UNDERSTANDING

THE EQUINE EYE

YOUR **GUIDE** TO HORSE HEALTH
CARE AND MANAGEMENT

D1598488

Copyright © 1999 The Blood-Horse, Inc.

All Rights reserved. No part of this book may be repro-
duced in any form by any means, including photocopying,
audio recording, or any information storage or retrieval system, without the permission in writing from the copyright
holder. Inquiries should be addressed to Publisher, The
Blood-Horse, Inc., Box 4038, Lexington, KY 40544-4038.

ISBN 1-58150-032-7

Printed in the United States of America

UNDERSTANDING
THE EQUINE
EYE

YOUR **GUIDE** TO HORSE HEALTH
CARE AND MANAGEMENT

By Michael A. Ball, DVM

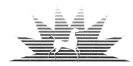

The Blood-Horse, Inc. Lexington, KY

Contents

DEDICATION

I would like to dedicate this book to Dr. William C. Rebhun, professor of large animal medicine and ophthalmology at Cornell University. Dr. Rebhun was a close friend, professional colleague, and mentor for many years. While I was a veterinary student at Cornell, Dr. Rebhun became one of my most influential mentors due to his extreme professionalism and profound diagnostic skills as a veterinarian. His compassion for the animals he cared for and his enthusiasm for teaching veterinary students and residents was always outstanding.

As I pursued my career as a veterinarian, Dr. Rebhun and I shared many clinical cases and worked together on research developing new treatments for ophthalmic diseases. Dr. Rebhun was instrumental in my development as a veterinarian and the passion I have for conditions involving the horse's eye.

INTRODUCTION

As far back as equine literature exists, eyes have been viewed by many as windows to the horse's soul, to its ability to perform and understand, even an indication of how much "heart" it has. Bright, kind or intelligent eyes have influenced more than one sale.

There is no scientific research to support such ideas, but it IS true that the eye is a source of wonder and beauty.

The way it collects light and transfers light signals to the brain to form an image is a fascinating scientific process. It is also a complex process involving the physics of lenses as the eye bends and focuses light. That triggers a complex series of biochemical reactions, which create nerve impulses that are sent to the brain.

The equine eye and vision present challenging questions because the horse cannot tell us what it sees. What does that jump look like as a horse approaches it? What do humans look like to the horse? Do horses need glasses?

In *Understanding the Equine Eye*, we will look at some of the research on how horses see and perceive their world. We also will review the anatomy of the eye, vision testing and examination, and common equine eye diseases such as conjunctivitis and uveitis. The book also will discuss when you should call the veterinarian and what you, the owner or manager, should and should not do when your horse is suffering from an eye problem or injury.

Although much remains unknown about equine vision, understanding and putting to good use the available information and data can help us as caretakers ensure the health and well-being of our equine friends and their bright orbs.

Michael A. Ball, DVM
Cornell University
Ithaca, New York

CHAPTER 1

Anatomy of the Equine Eye

T he equine eye is a symphony with many parts working in concert to create the end result: vision. Each part is susceptible to disease. To understand those diseases and how they can affect vision, it is important to know the structure and function of the parts.

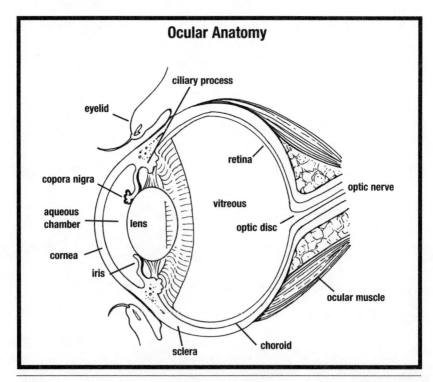

Ocular Anatomy

ciliary process

eyelid

retina

copora nigra

optic nerve

aqueous chamber

vitreous

lens

optic disc

cornea

iris

ocular muscle

sclera

choroid

THE EYELIDS

The eyelids include the eyelashes and surrounding longer tactile hairs. In a sense, the lashes are the first line of defense in protecting the eye.

The lashes are extremely sensitive and can trigger a lightning-fast blink reflex, slamming the eyelids shut to ward off incoming danger that could cut the cornea or eyelid. (For that reason, the lashes and other tactile eye hairs should not be trimmed for cosmetic purposes. If the longer hairs cannot be left long on that blue-ribbon conformation hunter, they should never be cut back all the way — leave at least 1 inch of hair intact.)

> ## AT A GLANCE
>
> • The horse is one of just a few species which have a third eyelid; it acts like a windshield wiper.
>
> • The lachrimal glands produce tears and keep the surface of the cornea from drying out.
>
> • The cornea can be likened to an onion because of its many layers.

The eyelids contain numerous muscles that are both fast and strong; just ask anyone who has tried to pry apart a horse's lids to apply medication. The eyelids also continuously distribute tear film that wipes away dirt and debris that enter the eye. Eyelid lacerations are fairly common and will be discussed in more detail later.

THE "THIRD" EYELID

The third eyelid is a structure limited to horses and a few other species. Barely visible when the eye is open, it sits under the eye in the medial canthus. The corners of the eye are called the canthus, with medial being toward the nose (or nasal) and lateral being on the outside (or temporal).

The third eyelid is a mass of soft tissue with a T-shaped piece of cartilage imbedded deep within it. It sweeps across the surface of the eye when the lids blink, acting like a windshield wiper to remove dust and debris and spreading the tear film across the corneal surface.

The third eyelid is a common location for "cancer eye,"

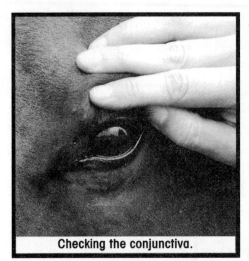
Checking the conjunctiva.

which will be discussed later. Foreign objects also can become lodged in the soft tissue of the third eyelid, causing chronic irritation and ulceration of the cornea.

THE CONJUNCTIVA

The conjunctiva is the soft pink tissue lining the undersides of the eyelids and covering the third eyelid. The conjunctiva is rich in lymph tissue (tissue of the immune system) and blood supply. Inflammation of the conjunctiva is called conjunctivitis — a problem familiar to all allergy sufferers.

The conjunctiva adds a protective substance to the surrounding tissue of the eye. But foreign objects can become lodged here and cause chronic irritation or ulceration of the cornea.

It is important to note that the surface of the eye and the surrounding tissue are not a sterile environment. A culture grown from the surface of the cornea will show a number of bacterial, fungal, and yeast organisms. That is normal. The system of defense mechanisms, such as tears, keeps these organisms in check and prevents disease.

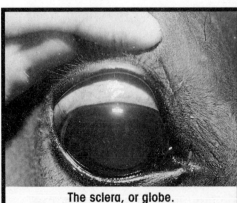
The sclera, or globe.

THE SCLERA

The sclera is the white part of the eyeball, or the globe. Strong tissue forms 75% of the sclera. Blood vessels can enter the sclera during inflammations, and this is the part of the eye that becomes "bloodshot." The development of such blood vessels can be a sign of numerous diseases. The sclera is also the part of the eye that becomes yellow due to jaundice (icterus), a sign of liver disease, or lack of appetite.

The sclera is also the structure to which all muscles responsible for movement of the globe connect.

THE LACHRIMAL GLANDS

The lachrimal glands produce tears. Tear film is extremely important for the eye's health and well-being.

Tear film consists of three separate layers only a fraction of a millimeter thick. The film's inner portion is designed to stick to the surface of the cornea and provide moisture and protection. The outer layer has a lipid-type chemical composition to prevent rapid evaporation when the eye is open. The tear film also contains chemicals that work in the eye's immune system.

Without tear film, the surface of the cornea will become dry and predisposed to chronic ulcers or sores. There is a condition in dogs in which decreased production of tear film leads to "dry eye." These dogs suffer from chronic ulcers. This condition occasionally occurs in the horse and can be a side effect of several commonly used pharmaceuticals.

THE LACHRIMAL DUCTS/PUNCTA

Tears wash away debris that collects on the surface of the eye. With help from the eyelid, the debris is "flushed" away through the tear ducts.

In the medial canthus area are two openings called "puncta." They drain into the lachrimal duct (or nasolacrimal duct), which travels in the skull along the facial crest toward the nose. The duct opens about 3 inches inside the nostril on the outer aspect. If you look up the outer aspect of your horse's nose with a flashlight, you will see a small pink hole — this is where tears from the eye drain. That is one of the reasons why you will see a veterinarian use a bright yellow ulcer stain on a horse's eye. If all is well, the stain will come out the nostril.

A blockage of the nasolacrimal duct will lead to a chronically "runny" eye (to be discussed later).

THE EXTRAOCULAR MUSCLES

Behind the eye are a series of muscles that coordinate the movement of the eye in all directions. The muscles are controlled by cranial nerves (among the 12 major nerves that come directly from the brain and control various body functions).

With a neurologic disease, the abnormal position of the eye can indicate what part of the brain is affected by the problem. In addition, the rapid, repetitive vertical or horizontal movement of the eye (nystagmus) can provide clues about the origins of certain neurologic diseases.

THE CORNEA

I often liken the cornea to a slice of onion because it is comprised of many layers made up of different structures.

The cornea is the outer clear surface of the globe. It is very thin (about half a millimeter, the thickness of a fingernail) and is where many eye diseases occur. The cornea allows light into the back of the eye, but it also serves as the major focusing device.

The outer layer of the cornea is called the epithelium. The epithelium is a layer of cells that acts as a barrier to water, dirt, debris, and microorganisms. The epithelium is fat-soluble (or lipid-soluble), an important point when it comes to drug therapy. Water soluble drugs do not penetrate the barrier well, but fat, or lipid, soluble drugs do.

The middle layer is water soluble and is called the stroma. If there is a break in the epithelium because of a laceration, water from the tear film will enter and collect within the stroma, causing a buildup of fluid (edema).

The innermost layer is the endothelium and is extremely thin (one cell layer thick). The endothelium has a very important job — it keeps the cornea clear and transparent. Its biochemical function is to remove water from the middle layer and keep the cornea "dehydrated." When the cornea takes on water, the middle layer (stroma) becomes a cloudy white/blue and is less transparent. This is the classic appearance of corneal edema.

Corneal edema can come from a break in the epithelium or a problem with the endothelium. We will discuss specific causes of corneal edema later; for now it is important to know that the cornea's clarity is due to the relatively dehydrated state caused by the inner layer and maintained, in part, by the water-resistant outer layer.

Another important aspect of the cornea is that it is one of the few tissues in the body with no blood vessels. The corneal tissues get their oxygen from surface contact inside and outside.

The cornea's lack of blood supply places it at a disadvantage in fighting infection because many of the body's defense mechanisms travel to infected sites through the blood stream (antibodies, white blood cells, etc.). When the cornea is infected, blood vessels grow from the surrounding tissue to the surface of the cornea. But because of the time it takes for the vessels to grow (about 2 millimeters a day in a normal eye), this gives the disease an advantage. It is often a race to see whether the blood vessels can reach the infection soon enough.

THE ANTERIOR CHAMBER

Behind the cornea is a space known as the anterior (front) chamber. This space is between the inner surface of the cornea and the surface of the iris and lens. It is filled with fluid called aqueous humor. The fluid is clear so light can pass through on its way to the back of the eye.

The anterior chamber is where signs of periodic ophthalmia (uveitis or moon blindness) often are observed.

The aqueous humor is produced and drained from the chamber at a constant rate. If something goes wrong and fluid production decreases, the eye will "deflate" and become soft. Should fluid production become too great or fluid drainage decrease, the eye will develop glaucoma.

THE IRIS

The iris is typically brown tissue circling the black pupil (really the lens). This is the tissue that constricts or dilates the pupil depending on light intensity. The iris has a great number of blood vessels and is one of the primary tissues affected by uveitis or moon blindness.

THE NIGRA BODIES

It has been hypothesized that the nigra bodies function as an internal sun shade. These small dark "punching bag"-type structures are on the upper surface of the iris and are normal in the horse. They occasionally can be found on the lower border of the iris, but this is less common. Sometimes they become enlarged and form cystlike structures that can affect vision.

THE LENS

The lens is a soft structure that sits in the pupil and is normally clear. It can appear red on a photograph from the light of a camera flash (people) or bright yellow-green from a car's headlights (many animals).

From the posterior (back) surface of the lens there is a clear, jellylike substance called the vitreous, then the retina on the posterior part of the eye.

The lens focuses the light further onto the back of the eye, although not as much in the horse as in people. The cornea actually provides most of the focusing.

The lens does function as a true optical lens; as with a camera, it inverts the image so that when the image hits the back of the eye, it is upside down and backward. The brain puts the image back into the proper orientation.

The muscles that attach to the lens change its shape, allowing it to focus on objects at different distances. As the next chapter will discuss, this is much less crucial for the horse's ability to focus on far/near objects than it is for people.

If the lens becomes opaque, it is considered a cataract.

THE POSTERIOR CHAMBER

The chamber between the back of the lens and the retina (back of the eye) is filled with another clear fluid (the vitreous humor) that is slightly thicker than the anterior chamber fluid. This fluid gives more substance to the eye and holds the retina in place. It also protects the retina by acting as a shock absorber if there is any type of trauma to the eye.

THE RETINA

The retina is extremely complex, existing as layers of receptors that convert the light image focused on the back of the eye to an electrical signal that's transmitted to the brain.

Some of the major receptors are called rods and cones. They differ in their sensitivity to the brightness of light focused on the back of the eye. The ratio of these cells is what allows some animals to have better low-light vision than others. The greater the number of rods, the better the dim light vision.

This is also where color vision comes into play, with some cells (cones) being sensitive to different colors of the visible light spectrum. In some species, visual acuity is based on receptors that respond to wavelengths of light beyond the spectrum visible to humans (infrared).

THE TEPEDUM

The tepedum is a highly reflective layer of cells in the upper portion of the back of the eye. It is the structure responsible for those eerie yellow spots you see on the side of the road when you drive home late at night.

These cells collect and amplify light to enhance low-light

vision. In the horse, this layer can be seen as a beautiful green-ish/yellow color reflecting in the upper portion of the back of the eye. To get a good look, go out in the barn at night and leave the lights off. Use a pen light and hold the horse's head slightly elevated. Shine the light into the back of the horse's eye. The greenish/yellow reflection is the tepedum.

THE CHOROID

The choroid is the structure that sits on the sclera at the very back of the eye. It serves as the major blood supply to the retina. In pigmented breeds (horses with black skin), this layer will be dark brown; in non-pigmented breeds (white-skinned horses), it will be bright red because you will see the blood vessels. This is why the eyes of some white-faced horses will reflect red when you shine a light in the back of the eyes.

Humans don't have a tepedum or pigmented tissue, which is why human eyes are red in some photographs.

THE OPTIC NERVE

The optic nerve can be seen as a yellow/white disc slightly below the center of the back of the eye. The disc is different in all species of animals. All but the horse have relatively large blood vessels near the disc. The horse has hundreds of very fine blood vessels radiating from the perimeter of the disc, looking almost like a beautiful sunset. The disc is the end of the optic nerve and transmits all visual data to the brain.

THE OPTIC CHIASM

The optic chiasm is where the two optic nerves come to-gether and cross over. It sits just under the pituitary gland on the floor of the brain. The crossover is not unique to the horse. It is where much of the information from the right eye is sent to the left side of the brain, and vice versa.

THE OPTIC CORTEX

This is in the frontal lobe of the brain, where the information being transmitted from the eye is finally perceived as an image. Again, the right side of the brain is processing much of the information from the left eye, and vice versa.

CHAPTER 2

How the Horse Sees

Theories and controversy about how a horse perceives its world have existed for more than a century. The main questions are these:

1. Does a horse bring a visual image into focus using the eye's lens, as people do, or by moving its head?

2. Does a horse see in color?

3. Do horses suffer from visual defects such as nearsightedness (myopia) or farsightedness (hyperopia) that might affect performance?

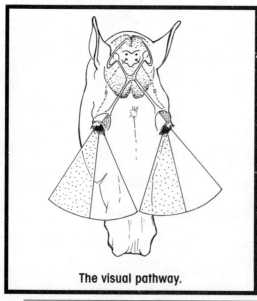

The visual pathway.

Whatever the answers, normal vision is very important to the horse's daily life. As the late James Law, a professor of veterinary science at Cornell University, said in a 1923 edition of a U.S. Department of Agriculture Special Report of Diseases of the Horse: "We can scarcely overestimate the value of sound eyes in the horse, and hence all the diseases and injuries which seriously interfere with vision are matters of extreme gravity and apprehension … as a mere matter of beauty, a sound, full, clear, intelligent eye is something which must always add a high value to our equine friends and servants."

At its essence, the visual system collects light and focuses it on the retina in the back of the eye, where the image is transmitted to the brain via the nervous system. The point at which the light, and hence the image, is focused on the retina functions very much like a camera lens. In people and domestic animals, small muscles can change the shape of the lens (the soft structure behind the pupil). This change brings an image into focus on the retina. If the image is not in focus, then the image perceived by the brain is not in focus — time for glasses or contact lenses.

The equine eye has the largest globe of all land mammals. The subsequent increase in retinal area allows for a relative image magnification 50% greater than that of the human eye. Based on physics, this means there is the potential for the horse to perceive things 50% larger than we do. But we do not know whether a 5-foot jump

AT A GLANCE

- The equine eye has the largest globe of all land mammals.

- It is possible that horses see objects 50% larger than humans do, but no one really knows.

- The horse has an amazing 350 degrees of total visual field.

- It is thought that horses might raise and lower their heads to focus on objects.

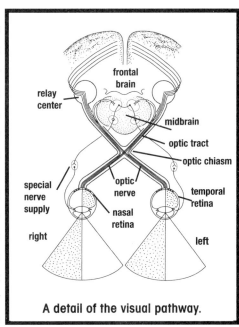

A detail of the visual pathway.

looks 7½ feet tall to the horse. The horse's eyes are set out laterally from the skull and protrude farther forward than the human eye. This placement allows for an exceptional field of vision; the horse can see 190 to 195 degrees horizontally and about 175 degrees vertically. The horse has an amazing 350 degrees of total visual field, with a narrow blind spot immediately in front of the nose and another blind spot a few meters behind the rump. Where a horse directs its ears has been purported to reflect the direction in which it is focusing its vision.

Vision is considered monocular or binocular. Humans are binocular, meaning each eye covers part of the other's field of vision. In a monocular species, each eye does its own thing and does not share any part of the visual field with the other eye. The horse has about 65% crossover vision and is therefore somewhat binocular.

THE RAMPED RETINA THEORY

The "ramped retina" controversy started in 1930.

Because the equine lens is unable to change shape that

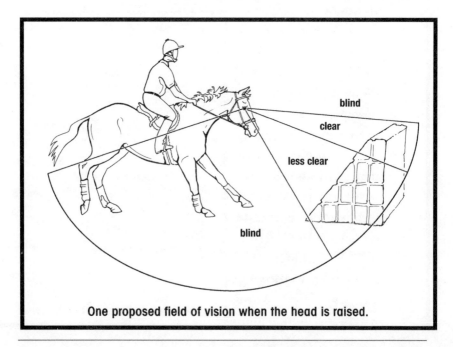

One proposed field of vision when the head is raised.

well, it might not be the sole mechanism of focusing light on the retina. It was proposed in 1930, 1942, and 1960 by independent researchers that the retina — and hence the back of the equine eye — is not perfectly round, but sloped or "ramped." This means the horse might be able, by raising or lowering its head, to "find" a retinal location where the light is in focus. A 1975 study failed to back the findings, but a 1977 study supported the idea that a horse might have to move its head, eye, or both for optimal visual acuity. It is generally believed that the horse must elevate its head to "focus" on objects close by and lower its head to focus on more distant objects.

As with many other finer details of equine vision, the ramped retina theory is still somewhat controversial. It is likely that focusing requires use of the lens and head movement. In my experience, when the head is restricted, horses often display actions that might indicate poor visual acuity, such as head shaking and shying away from objects, imaginary or otherwise.

Visual acuity is basically image resolution and is deter-

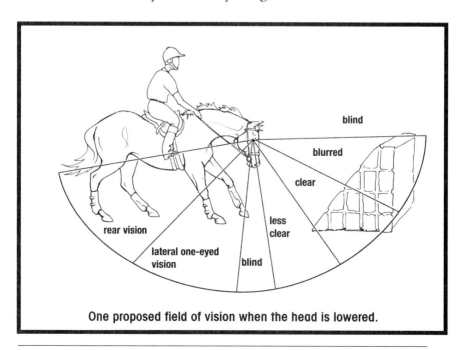

One proposed field of vision when the head is lowered.

mined by numerous factors, including the type and density of photoreceptor cells; details of the nervous tissue in the retina; and things that affect light as it passes through the eye, such as pupil size.

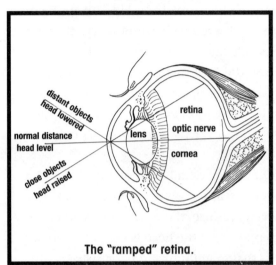

The "ramped" retina.

Visual acuity in the horse and how it compares to other species are based on estimates. The horse is estimated to have 0.6 of the visual acuity of humans. So if a person has 20/20 vision, a horse would be expected to have about 20/33. That means an object a person sees from 33 feet away looks 20 feet away to the horse. The horse is estimated to have three times the visual acuity of cats.

COULD A HORSE NEED GLASSES?

A report from the American Museum of Natural History in 1961 indicated that some domesticated horses are nearsighted. Myopia is an error of refraction in which light entering the eye parallel to the optic axis is brought into focus in front of the retina. This results in a blurred image.

But if the horse does have a ramped retina, it might be able to raise or lower the head until the image is in focus. This, of course, is speculation, and how an image is perceived by the horse's brain as it gazes out from a summer pasture probably will remain a mystery.

CAN HORSES SEE IN COLOR?

The horse's retina does have the type of photoreceptor cell needed for color vision (the so-called "cone" cell). This is another controversial topic for which we probably will never know the answer.

Horses are thought to have some color vision and, based on some reports, respond best to yellow, followed by green and blue. Red is thought to be more difficult for them to see. Interestingly, one study that correlated the color of jump rails to the frequency of knocked-down rails indicated that yellow jump rails were knocked down most often.

CHAPTER 3

Examination of the Equine Eye

"Have you noticed any changes in your vision?"

"Yes. In fact, I'm starting to have trouble reading the street signs while driving."

"Well then, sit back and relax. I'm going to dim the lights and have you read the letters as you look through the machine. Which letter is sharper? This one or this one? This one or this one?"

Sound familiar? For those of you who wear glasses, this is a routine visit to the optometrist.

"Have you noticed any changes in your vision?"

"Yes. In fact, I'm starting to have trouble seeing the jumps, especially at dusk. I also have been bumping into the pasture fence more that usual."

"Well then, stand there and relax. I'm going to dim the lights and have you read the images while you look through the machine. Which carrot is sharper? This one or this one? This one or this one?"

Unfortunately, this conversation will never happen. There are no machines to test a horse's vision, and a horse cannot tell the examiner what it sees.

Vision testing in horses is not an exact science. The main

goal of the ophthalmic examination is to identify abnormalities and speculate how they could affect vision based on known structure and function of the eye. Obviously, if there is a large, dense scar on the cornea from a previous infection or a very dense cataract, vision will be affected. The challenge occurs in trying to determine when smaller lesions affect total vision.

The examination starts with historical information. Is the horse headshy even when no behavior modification tech-

AT A GLANCE

• The main goal of an eye exam is to identify abnormalities and speculate how they could affect vision.

• An eye exam starts with historical information.

• A "menace" test is an important part of the exam.

• A veterinarian will use a penlight and an ophthalmoscope to evaluate the eyes.

niques are being used, such as smacking in the muzzle for frequent biting? Does the horse have a "sidedness" to the head-shyness, i.e., only when someone or something is on a particular side of the horse? Does the horse exhibit similar behavior when turned out in pasture, free in the stall or being worked? Has there been any head trauma — hitting the trailer or starting gate, being kicked, or flipping over on the cross-ties?

The next step is to stand back and look at the horse. Is there anything abnormal about the appearance of the eyes? Are they symmetrical? Does the horse have any scars or fresh wounds on one side of the head that could indicate it frequently bumps into things on that side? If there are positive historical or general examination findings, it could raise suspicions of a visual deficit.

This first part of the vision test is called the "menace." It is just that. A menacing hand gesture is made toward the horse's eye to see whether it will blink. This must be done carefully so 1) the other eye cannot see the movement and 2) the hand motion does not touch the lashes or create a strong enough air current to be felt, both of which will make the horse blink. Obviously, if the horse is blind or has significant visual impairment, it will not blink. But if there is a partial blind spot, the degree of impairment cannot be assessed very well in this manner.

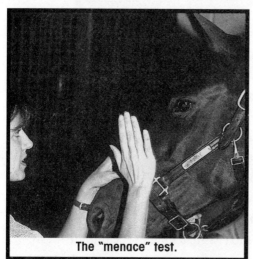
The "menace" test.

As the test continues, a veterinarian uses two common instruments to assess the equine eye: a penlight or other strong focal light and an ophthalmoscope. The eye is evaluated using a systematic approach that looks for corneal scars, and abnormalities in the anterior chamber, iris, or lens.

Corneal scars are the result of previous infection or trauma. Depending on the cause, scars can be as small as a pinhead or cover most of the cornea. If small, they probably don't affect vision significantly. As one would assume, the larger the scar, the greater the chance of it affecting vision.

On rare occasions, cysts on the iris can be seen hanging over the pupil like small punching bags. If large enough, these cysts can obstruct the pupil and actually move in the aqueous humor, creating a moving "shadow" or visual deficit to which the horse might react adversely. In some horses that have had an inflamed anterior chamber (infection, uveitis), the iris can form an adhesion to the surface of the lens. These horses might be unable to dilate their pupils in low light. In some cases, the adhesion can be significant enough to obstruct the pupil.

Cataracts, although rare in adult horses, are usually secondary to a prior ocular trauma or chronic uveitis and can obstruct the flow of light through the eye, affecting vision. The larger and more dense the cataract, the greater chance it will harm vision.

The ophthalmoscope is used to evaluate the fundus (back of the eye). With magnification of 15 times, it can check the health of the optic nerve and the remainder of the fundus for scars. Eyes that have suffered from uveitis or other severe ocular inflammations can develop scar tissue,

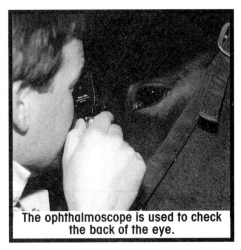

The ophthalmoscope is used to check the back of the eye.

leading to dysfunctional retinal areas in the fundus. These scarred areas can be related to blind spots, and the larger the scars the greater the chance of a significant effect on vision.

A more unusual and infrequent finding in the fundus is a "vitreal floater." Sometimes after a serious inflammation in the back of the eye, the vitreous humor becomes more liquid, and small collections of inflammatory debris can "float" around. These vitreal floaters, if large enough, could disrupt the visual field when a horse moves its head, thus causing it to spook, but the true relationship between the floater and behavior is unknown.

What if, upon inspection, the horse seems normal but is blind? This is where history might be helpful. With some head trauma, the optic nerve, not the eye, has been damaged. It can take several weeks or longer for the damage to become apparent in a fundic examination.

Other non-ocular causes for blindness should be evaluated as well. More discussion about such non-ocular abnormalities will follow.

CHAPTER 4

Ocular Diseases

SEVERE ACUTE OCULAR PAIN

Any degree of ocular pain should be considered an emergency until the cause has been identified. The signs of ocular pain are squinting, tearing, a pupil that's too small for the amount of ambient light, and an increased sensitivity to light. Ocular pain in the horse can be caused by many things, but common reasons are a scratch or developing ulcer on the cornea, or uveitis (moon blindness).

In many cases, the horse will not allow an exam without veterinary assistance because of the pain and because of its strong upper eyelid muscle. The horse often will need to be sedated and given a local anesthetic to paralyze the upper eyelid to aid in the examination.

It is important to seek veterinary care relatively quickly. If there is a scratch or ulcer, it must be determined whether the cause is a foreign body, such as a splinter or plant material, that is stuck in the conjunctiva or third eyelid. If a foreign object is not removed quickly, the ulcer

Squinting can be a sign of ocular pain.

will worsen. A foreign body in the cornea also needs to be removed as quickly as possible.

The eye is not a sterile environment. If the conjunctiva is cultured, a number of bacterial and fungal organisms can be grown, all of which can infect an abrasion, scratch, or ulcer. In addition, most foreign bodies that commonly end up in the horse eye are plant material or dirt, which have high contamination potential.

AT A GLANCE

- Signs of ocular pain include squinting, tearing, and increased sensitivity to light.

- Uveitis is a painful and sometimes recurring condition which can be caused by trauma, infection, and other factors.

- A variety of organisms can cause fungal infections.

One extremely important thing NOT to do is to put eye ointment from another horse, small animal, or yourself in a horse with a runny, painful eye. Using an inappropriate ointment can have devastating consequences. Ointments containing steroids have been associated with severe fungal eye disease in horses.

For comfort, a horse with a painful eye should be placed in a dark stall and be seen by a veterinarian as soon as possible. In most cases involving ulcers, treatment should not be complicated, but because some infections can be "fast and furious," particularly *Pseudomonas* and fungal infections, extra concern is warranted for a horse with a painful eye.

PERIODIC OPHTHALMIA

Periodic ophthalmia, otherwise known as recurrent uveitis (pronounced U-V-itis), uveitis, or moon blindness, can be devastating. Beyond that, little is known despite research over the years. (The term moon blindness comes from the ancient belief that the disease was associated with changes in the lunar

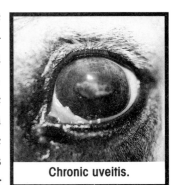

Chronic uveitis.

cycle. The "recurrent" reference stems from the fact that the disease has a propensity to recur unpredictably after the first occurrence.)

Uveitis is an inflammation of the uvea, which includes most of the interior parts of the eye that have a large blood supply. This is especially true for the iris or colored part of the eye surrounding the pupil.

The suspected causes

Uveitis can result from anything that causes inflammation in the eye and does not necessarily have to be associated with recurrent uveitis. Trauma to the eye, such as being hit with a polo ball, can induce uveitis. If the trauma involves a wound of any sort, then uveitis can be caused by infection. If a corneal ulcer caused by bacteria, fungi, or yeast becomes severe enough and starts to involve the deeper layer of the cornea, it can induce uveitis. Sometimes these corneal infections can rupture into the anterior chamber and cause very severe uveitis. In addition, severe systemic infection (most typically neonatal septicemia) can have a uveitis component; the presence of uveitis in a neonate can indicate a systemic disease.

Suspected causes of recurrent uveitis or periodic ophthalmia include the bacteria *Leptospira* and *Streptococcus equi* (the cause of strangles) and the parasite *Onchocerca cervicali*. The most common explanations for inflammation of the uvea are delayed hypersensitivity reaction and an autoimmune-mediated phenomenon.

Delayed hypersensitivity reaction is one of four classic immune responses to a foreign substance in the body. Essentially, an autoimmune-mediated reaction develops after exposure to a foreign substance. Some of the immune cells "remember" the foreign substance and are thought to remain on the uveal tissue. When the horse (and subsequently the immune cells) are exposed to the same foreign substance again, the reaction stimulates inflammation.

The autoimmune phenomenon occurs when the immune

system, for whatever reason, stops recognizing part of the body and starts to reject it. After a horse is infected with one of the causes of recurrent uveitis, the body may produce immunoproteins (antibodies) that target the uveal tissue. This could occur if the protein structure of part of the infectious agent is similar to the protein structure of part of the uveal tissue. A classic human example is rheumatic fever; the heart valves are attacked by the immune system after infection with the bacteria that causes strep throat.

Clinical signs

The primary sign of uveitis is pain manifested by squinting, tearing, and greater sensitivity to light. Other signs include a very constricted pupil (even in a dark stall), cloudiness within the eye (it will be difficult to see the iris and pupil, and there is a distinct haze), and the presence of solid material (protein) attached to the iris. Here is how that happens:

As the inflammation occurs, irritating chemicals are produced and released into the fluid in the anterior chamber (the space filled with a clear fluid between the inside of the cornea and the iris). In addition, white blood cells and protein leak from the inflamed blood vessels into the anterior chamber fluid, creating the haze in the anterior chamber. In severe cases of uveitis, the white blood cells will settle and collect in the floor of the anterior chamber. One of the proteins that leaks into the anterior chamber is called fibrin. Fibrin is a light, fluffy, cotton candy-like substance that is a precursor to a dense, connective tissue scar. If fibrin production is heavy and goes without treatment, it can cause a significant amount of scarring. Matured fibrin can glue the iris to the lens, thus preventing it from opening in low light, or it can cover the lens and greatly affect vision. An untreated inflammation can have a devastating effect on vision.

The signs of prior uveitis can be more subtle and require extensive examination of the outer and inner areas of the eye. This is an important part of any pre-purchase examination because of the recurrent nature of uveitis. Unfortunately, it is impossible for a veterinarian to predict whether the uveitis will recur. All a veterinarian can do is try to determine how the damage affects vision and document the extent of the lesions.

The most subtle sign of prior uveitis is a darkening of the iris, to a dark chocolate color, without obvious scarring of the iris. In advanced cases, the iris can appear moth-eaten and scarred. The edge of the iris might be irregular and roughened. (Remember, the little "punching bags" on the iris — nigra bodies — are normal.) Also, the surface of the lens (within the pupil area) might have a piece of iris, the iris itself or scar tissue stuck to it from the previous inflammation. Sometimes there are white strands of scar tissue darting about inside the anterior chamber.

The most crucial aspect of the pre-purchase examination is deep inside the eye. It is possible not to have other telltale signs but to have significant scarring in the back of the eye. The lesions caused by uveitis in the back of the eye (where the light-sensing retina is) are reflective scars surrounding the optic disk (optic nerve as it enters the eye). These lesions are referred to as "butterfly" lesions because of their shape. Scarring in the back of the eye, depending on the degree, can cause a visual deficit or blind spot.

In more chronic cases of uveitis, the iris can become very scarred and light; the border of the iris can be irregular and glued to the lens; the lens can become opaque because of a cataract; the eye can be abnormally large and firm or small and soft; and vision could be severely impaired. Also in advanced cases, the cornea might not be healthy and could have an ulcer. In all cases, one or both eyes could be affected.

Treatment

Before initiating treatment for uveitis, it is imperative that a veterinarian make the diagnosis and evaluate the cornea for the presence of an ulcer. The two main drugs used to treat uveitis are atropine and corticosteroids.

Atropine serves several important purposes. It works by paralyzing some of the muscles of the iris, thus stopping the painful spasm and allowing the pupil to dilate. Dilation is very important; if the pupil remains constricted and in contact with much of the lens, the odds increase for the iris to become scarred to the lens. If atropine does not dilate the pupil, a dilation drug will be used.

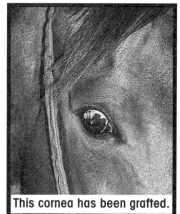

This cornea has been grafted.

Corticosteroids are potent anti-inflammatory drugs that typically are necessary to reduce inflammation. Corticosteroids are not risk-free. Because of their potent immune-suppressing abilities, corticosteroids, if used on an eye that has a corneal ulcer, can lead to a fungal eye infection. That happens in about 65% of horses treated with topical corticosteroids. Despite this risk, corticosteroids are necessary to control the inflammation associated with uveitis.

In addition to these two main treatments, topical antibiotics, topical antifungals, and topical non-steroidal anti-inflammatories are used. Systemic pain medication often is necessary, too.

There also is a rather neat (but expensive) treatment of high fibrin content in the anterior chamber. The greater the fibrin content, the greater the chance of permanent scarring and visual deficit. A drug called TPA (tissue plasminogen activator), used as a clot buster in human heart attack and stroke patients, can be injected into the eye to dissolve the fibrin.

Another potential treatment for advanced cases is the corneal grafting technique in which a cornea from a euthanized horse is transplanted on the affected horse's cornea.

Removing a severely infected eye (enucleation) is another option. This can be a very difficult decision, but sometimes it is the best option for the horse. An eye with chronic uveitis can be painful and require substantial treatment that results only in marginal comfort and does not save vision. Until there is a breakthrough in prevention or treatment, uveitis will remain the leading cause of blindness in horses.

FUNGAL EYE INFECTION

Fungal or mycotic keratitis (keratomycosis) is a well-known and frustrating clinical problem that was first described in people in 1879 and in the horse in 1973. Under the best of circumstances, the disease often requires prolonged and expensive treatment; at its worst, it can result in blindness or the need to remove the eye. In one review, 56% of equine keratomycosis cases had intact vision after treatment and 22% were enucleated, with nearly a third of those because of monetary constraints on the owners.

Fungal keratitis accounted for a quarter to more than one-third of the cases of infectious keratitis at three referral centers (University of Georgia, 33%; University of Missouri, 39%; and Cornell University, 22%). The clinical signs and currently available treatment options for keratomycosis have been extensively reported and reviewed in the literature.

Horses not only live in environments that harbor large numbers of fungal agents, but they frequently have fungal organisms in their conjunctivas. In addition, corneal injuries in horses often are caused by plant material or soil, either of which could be the source of a fungal infection. A multitude of causative fungal agents have been isolated from corneal infections in horses.

Although fungal keratitis has occurred sporadically in other species, horses frequently develop it, especially after inappropriate treatment of corneal epithelial defects with corticosteroids. (Remember, don't put ointments in the eye without veterinary consultation.) Topical corticosteroid treatment preceded referral in about 65% of keratomycosis cases reported in the veterinary literature.

Fungal pathogens that infect the equine cornea are usually opportunistic filamentous fungi or yeast organisms that reproduce by budding. The majority of filamentous organisms are septate hyphae forms and *Aspergillus* species and *Fusarium* species. *Dematiaceous* organisms such as *Alternaria* species and *Culveria* species are other occasionally isolated filamentous organisms. *Candida* species are the most common budding fungi to infect the human cornea.

Treatment

Like bacteria, fungal organisms have great species variances in pathologic mechanisms, metabolisms and toxin production, as well as growth requirements and susceptibility to antifungal drugs. Therefore, treatment for equine patients with fungal keratitis tends to be based on experience with previous cases, a limited number of currently available therapies, and, in many cases, economics.

The available topical medications have been reviewed extensively and repeatedly in the horse and people. These drugs usually are polyenes such as Natamycin and amphotericin B, or imidazoles (miconazole, clotrimazole, fluconazole, ketoconazole, and econazole) that bind with ergosterol (the essential chemical in fungal composition — similar to cholesterol in mammals) in the fungal cell membrane (polyenes) or inhibit ergosterol synthesis and possibly cause damage to the fungal cell wall. Miconazole is a common treatment using an intravenous solution ophthalmically. Miconazole was shown in 1988 to be highly efficacious (100% susceptibility against *Aspergillus* and *Fusarium*) but to have poor tissue penetration through intact rabbit corneal epithelium.

Natamycin is the only commercially produced ophthalmic approved for use in man and is the drug of choice for human fungal keratitis, especially in geographic areas where Fusarium species are the most common. Silver sulfadiazine also has been used alone or in combination with polyenes or imidazoles for the topical treatment of fungal keratitis, and it has proven antifungal activity.

Systemic therapy with imidazoles, alone or in combination

with topical medication, has been used in man to treat fungal keratitis with varying success. Similarly, some veterinarians, including myself, have used systemic imidazoles, such as ketoconazole (very expensive), in conjunction with ophthalmic antifungals when treating some extremely valuable animals. The systemic absorption of ketoconazole has been shown to be extremely poor in the horse, and there is no equine absorption data available for most others.

Itraconazole is a new antifungal compound that is highly lipophilic (likes fat tissue and therefore should penetrate the cornea wall). Itraconazole is thought to have greater antifungal activity than many of the previously available antifungal drugs. Itraconazole has been demonstrated to have a broad range of activity against various fungal species. Systemic treatment of fungal eye disease has been reported in people; there was a 55% cure rate with daily oral administration of itraconazole for 17 days, although this approach would be cost prohibitive for most equine cases.

A 1% itraconazole/30% DMSO petroleum-based topical ointment (developed by my research) has been shown to yield corneal concentrations of itraconazole up to 20 times the minimum concentration needed to inhibit growth for some species of *Aspergillus* and within the therapeutic range for *Fusarium* species when administered every six hours in the horse eye.

"CANCER" EYE

Cancer in the eye is one of the more common forms of cancer in the horse. The main form it takes is squamous cell carcinoma. Horses with white or non-pigmented skin surrounding the eye are at greatest risk. In addition, the Appaloosa appears to be predisposed to this problem, but it is seen in males and females of all breeds and ages.

As in people, the chance of getting such a tumor increases if the skin is exposed to lots of sunlight. The tumor most commonly affects the third eyelid, the junction between the white sclera and the cornea, and less commonly the margin of the eyelids. Such tumors have various looks to them; they often start as small, smooth lumps that go unnoticed until they start to look like warts with crumbly tissue that bleeds easily.

Because this tumor commonly develops in the third eyelid, it usually is hidden from view. So if a third eyelid becomes more prominent than the other, it could be a warning sign. Other signs include pain and chronic ocular discharge.

In their early stages, the lesions on the eyelids can be mistaken for sunburn, so the third eyelid must be pulled out and palpated. It is important to catch squamous cell carcinoma early, when the prognosis can be good. Typically, it is a slow-growing tumor that stays in one area, but it can invade surrounding tissue. If the tumor in the third eyelid moves into the skull, the prognosis is very poor.

If the tumor is confined to the third eyelid, the third eyelid is removed. The surgery is relatively simple and often can be performed at the farm under sedation and local anesthetic. If the tumor is on the eyeball, treatment usually involves surgical removal of the lesion followed by radiation therapy or freezing. Freezing, with liquid nitrogen, is a relatively successful way to kill these cancer cells.

If the lesion is on the eyelid, treatment can be difficult. If the lesion is surgically removed, it can be difficult to leave enough eyelid to function properly, so radiation therapy and freezing might be used.

OTHER CANCERS

There are forms of cancer that can affect the eye or surrounding tissue, but they are somewhat rare. Melanoma, the gray horse tumor, occasionally can affect the eye. I have seen melanomas in the surrounding ocular tissue, on the surface of the eye, inside the anterior chamber, and in the back of the eye. Other forms of cancer can affect all parts of the eye as well. Treatments are limited to chemotherapy, radiation therapy, and surgical removal of the affected tissue when possible.

CHAPTER 5

Eyelid Lacerations and Trauma

Foreign objects and blunt trauma can lacerate, puncture, or rupture the eye. The prognosis depends on the degree of damage and the amount of contamination or infection. To maximize the chances of a successful repair, the damaged eye should be examined immediately by a veterinarian. The more time that passes, the greater the chance of infection and complications.

Although many eyelid lacerations are small, they should be repaired if there is any chance they might permanently compromise the lid margins. Some corneal ulcers/trauma seem to occur near lid margin defects because the natural protection of the lids has been impaired.

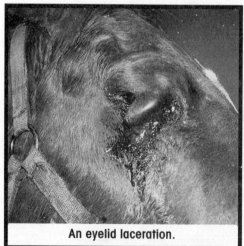

An eyelid laceration.

In many cases, it is extremely important for future eye health that lid lacerations be repaired correctly. If they are not, possible complications include chronic epiphora (ocular discharge), chronic conjunctivitis, exposure keratitis (inflammation of the cornea), recurrent corneal abrasions, and entropion (eyelashes that chronically irritate the cornea).

The first step in evaluating and repairing a lid laceration is sedation, so don't be alarmed if your veterinarian gives your horse a fairly heavy sedative. No one wants a horse to act up when a vet is holding a suture needle fractions of an inch from the animal's eye.

Many lacerations can be repaired on a standing horse under heavy sedation. An uncooperative horse might have to be anesthetized and laid down.

AT A GLANCE

- A damaged eye should be examined as quickly as possible by a veterinarian.

- Many eyelid lacerations warrant surgical repair to prevent future problems.

- Head trauma can trigger the development of uveitis and even blindness.

After sedation, the lid is anesthetized and paralyzed. Three to 4 ml of 2% lidocaine around the auriculopalpebral nerve as it crosses the zygomatic arch (this area can be palpated) will anesthetize the superior eye lid.

Anesthesia of all but the most lateral aspect of the superior lid is achieved by blocking the supraorbital nerve. This nerve can be palpated as the divot (supraorbital foramen) in the bony area just above the eye. It is a branch of the fifth cranial nerve (sensory) and produces regional anesthesia. Two to 3 ml of 2% lidocaine around the supraorbital nerve (over the divot) generally works well.

The lower lid and the most lateral (outer) aspect of the upper lid are served by the zygomatic and lacrimal nerves. Regional anesthesia cannot be performed in these areas, so a local anesthetic is necessary. Iodine-based surgical scrub is preferred because chlorhexidine (Nolvosan) has been shown to be toxic to corneal epithelium. Care should be taken to minimize a scrub solution's contact with the cornea; the cornea is usually protected by putting petroleum-based ointment on it.

After standard surgical preparation, the laceration is evaluated, and foreign bodies are removed. Even if the wound is 12 to 24 hours old, it should be repaired immediately. If more time has gone by and/or the wound appears to be significantly inflamed or infected, the laceration should not be surgically repaired until wound management and antibiotics have proven effective.

If performed carefully, a simple two-layer repair generally ensures functional and cosmetic results. The first layer of sutures is between the conjunctiva and skin in the lid stroma. Unless the conjunctiva is widely separated from the lid stroma, it generally does not require suturing.

The first suture is the most important and has to approximate the lid margin at the leading edge of the laceration. A good repair can greatly reduce complications by re-establishing continuity of the lid margin. Absorbable suture is used for the first layer, and great care should be taken, especially with the first suture, to ensure that no suture material or knot touches the cornea.

The second layer creates apposition of the skin and is a simple interrupted pattern with non-absorbable suture material. Again, great care should be taken to align the lid margin perfectly and ensure that no suture material touches the cornea. This layer is generally left in for 14 days to allow maximal tissue strength before removal.

After the lid has been repaired it is important to evaluate the eye for any abnormality. If significant trauma occurred with the laceration, it could lead to uveitis. The anterior chamber should be examined for aqueous flare or hyphema (blood in the anterior chamber) and the pupil for meiosis (pupillary dilation). If there are any signs of uveitis, appropriate treatment should begin. But care should be taken with topical corticosteroids because of: 1) their negative effects on wound healing and 2) the potential for increased risk of keratomycosis if corneal epithelial defects exist.

The cornea should be evaluated carefully for the presence of foreign bodies or epithelial defects. Fluorescein stain under an ultraviolet light (Wood's lamp) can greatly aid in identifying subtle corneal lesions. If a Wood's lamp is not available, a "black-light" bulb can function as an economical ultraviolet light source.

The use of topical antibiotics (triple-antibiotic, etc.) and systemic antibiotics (trimethoprim-sulfa or penicillin) are generally warranted for five to seven days after the repair. Also, the use of a systemic non-steroidal anti-inflammatory drug (phenylbutazone or flunixin meglumine) is beneficial for three to five days. And finally, tetanus toxoid should be given if necessary.

BLUNT OCULAR TRAUMA

Any type of accident or head injury could result in eye problems. I have seen eye injuries caused by trailer accidents, spooked horses that hit their heads on a wall or starting gate, and by polo balls and mallets. Although there might not be external damage such as a cut, there could be problems that are less evident.

For instance, blunt trauma can induce uveitis. If you know a horse has hit its head, the eyes should be evaluated for cloudiness or blood in the anterior chamber. The onset of this type of uveitis can be delayed or gradual, so the eyes should be monitored carefully for several days.

Blindness is another problem that can be caused by head trauma. If the force is hard and very sudden, the eye, which is relatively mobile in its socket, can move far enough and quickly enough to "snap" the optic nerve, causing swelling and damage. This type of injury is seen occasionally in people who hit their heads on steering wheels. The damage in horses is not always permanent; with prompt administration of anti-inflammatory drugs, the prognosis might improve.

CHAPTER 6

Enucleation

Enucleation (e-nuc-le-a-tion) basically means surgical removal of the eyeball. All the diseases that can result in blindness also might require removal of the eyeball. For most owners, this is an extremely difficult decision to make.

The procedure generally is reserved for cases in which the horse has lost the majority of viable vision and there is little hope of regaining it. In addition, the eye usually has become a chronic source of pain and discomfort.

If the eye must be removed, all is not always lost. In many

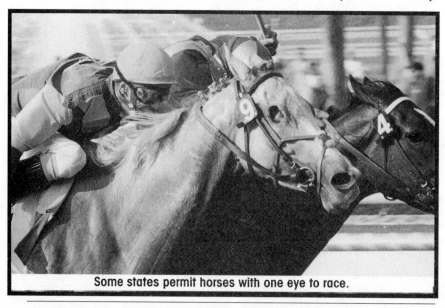

Some states permit horses with one eye to race.

states it is legal to race a horse that is blind on one side, and some show horse disciplines allow blindness in one eye.

The procedure generally requires general anesthesia, and the eye is removed using one of several procedures. Regardless of the removal method, the margins of the eyelids are sewn together. Immediately after surgery, the eye socket looks as if the eye is simply being held closed. With time, however, the blood clot behind the eyelids and the remaining tissue shrink, and a depression forms.

AT A GLANCE

- Enucleation is generally reserved for cases in which a horse has lost most of its vision.

- When a horse suffers chronic eye pain, enucleation might be in its best interest.

- Many horses still can lead useful and happy lives with one eye.

- Most horses have trouble dealing with total blindness.

Several procedures can be performed if cosmetic appearance is important. A prosthetic device (basically a sterile silicone ball) can be placed in the socket under the sutured lids to lessen the depression.

Another procedure works only when the injury is not infected and much of the eyeball is intact. This generally happens in cases

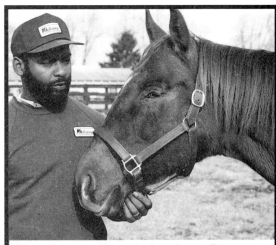

The well-known Kentucky broodmare Begum was a successful producer despite being blind.

of blunt trauma, such as a kick in the eye or getting hit with a polo ball or mallet. The eye is weakest at the junction between the cornea and the sclera, so a hard blow to the eye ruptures it along this margin. Vision cannot be restored, but a black silicon ball can be placed inside the eye so it looks as if the eye is intact

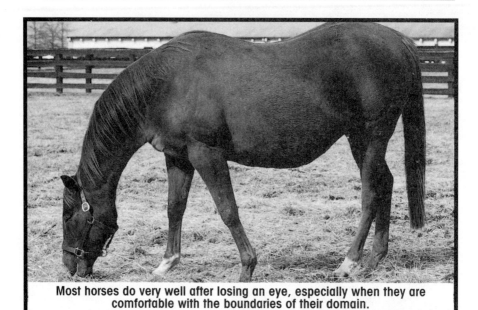

Most horses do very well after losing an eye, especially when they are comfortable with the boundaries of their domain.

with working lids. This operation is difficult and expensive and probably borders on unnecessary vanity, but it has been done.

By and large, most horses do very well after losing an eye. Their ability to compensate is truly remarkable. Of the 100-plus horses I know that had to have eyes removed, I cannot think of one that did not adjust quickly. Many of the horses had been experiencing chronic pain in the affected eyes and had limited vision, if any, before surgery; afterward, relief was almost immediate because the source of pain was gone.

When facing this situation, we must try to do what is best for the horse and keep our emotions somewhat under

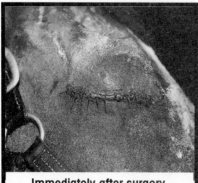

Immediately after surgery.

control (easier said than done). Most of the affected horses resumed performance careers if it was allowed or are living very comfortable lives.

One final note about removal: We must be certain to carefully evaluate the "good" eye, the one the horse will become dependent on, to make sure there are no problems there.

So what about the horse that is

blind in both eyes? This is a tough one, and most horses cannot deal with the situation. In addition, there is the ethical question about the quality of life for a blind horse. I know of several blind horses that have made excellent mothers. They are confined to an area with very safe fencing; they seem to have

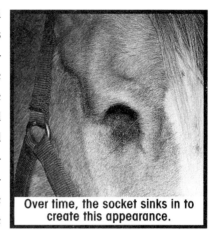

Over time, the socket sinks in to create this appearance.

learned the boundaries of their domain and lead what appear to be relatively happy lives. Their foals wear bells around their necks so they are easy to locate.

That appears to be the exception, however. Most blind horses are somewhat dangerous to be around.

CHAPTER 7

Miscellaneous Ocular Problems

CONJUNCTIVITIS

The term conjunctivitis means inflammation of the conjunctiva, the soft pink tissue surrounding the eye. The main clinical signs of conjunctivitis are ocular discharge, irritation or pain, and a reddening of the conjunctival tissue.

The term is a broad one and can be caused by a variety of problems. Many people suffer from conjunctivitis caused by allergies. Allergies possibly can trigger conjunctivitis in horses, but the diagnosis is often an assumed one. In dogs, goats, cows, and especially cats, there are several well-documented bacterial and viral causes for conjunctivitis. There is less evidence for such a cause in the horse, but a viral and bacterial cause probably does contribute to cases of equine conjunctivitis.

There are several systemic diseases that can cause the development of conjunctivitis, such as equine viral arteritis (EVA). In addition, conjunctival irritation by flies and chemicals such as fly spray can cause conjunctivitis. Most commonly, conjunctivitis is secondary to another ocular problem. It is important to have a horse with conjunctivitis evaluated by your veterinarian as it may be a more obvious sign of a less obvious (and more severe) problem.

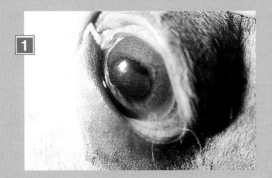

A foal with a small piece of wood imbedded in the cornea (photo 1); it was flushed out with sterile saline from a syringe; in photo 2, a foal with a small piece of hair imbedded in its eye, which caused an infection. The hair was removed surgically and the infected tissue debrided.

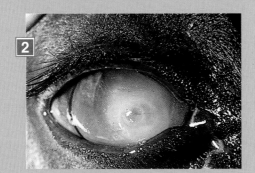

The horse in photo 3 has a "subpalpebral lavage system" in place for the application of medications to the eye. Note the prominent cataract.

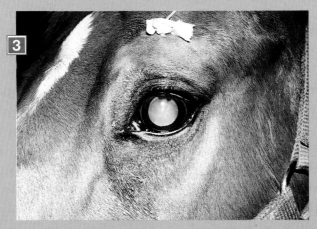

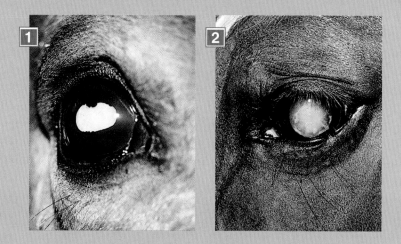

The horse in photo 1 has a prominent cataract as shown by the white opaqueness of the lens. On a normal pupil this is clear and dark; an older horse with a prominent cataract (photo 2). Note the light refracting back off the opaque part of the lens.

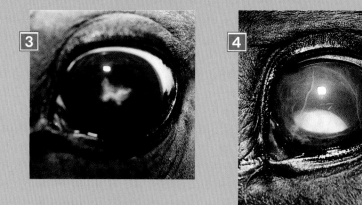

A butterfly-shaped cataract in the lens of an adult horse (photo 3). There was no known cause for its development. Photo 4 shows an eye with a prominent cataract, plus a lens which has been dislocated from the pupil. You can see the normal black pupil in the upper quadrant and the curve of the dislocated lens across the middle of the pupil. This particular case resulted from blunt trauma to the eye.

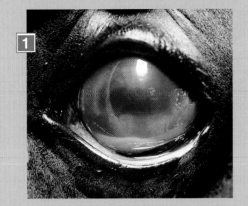

The eye in photo 1 has uveitis. There is haze in the anterior chamber, obscuring the iris, and a puddle of white blood cells in the chamber's lower portion; photo 2 shows a view of the back of the eye as seen with the aid of an ophthalmoscope. The circular pink structure in the center is the optic disc. The bright greenish/yellow portion above this is the tepedum licidum, the reflective cell that amplifies light. The white patch surrounding the optic disc is a scar that is characteristic of uveitis.

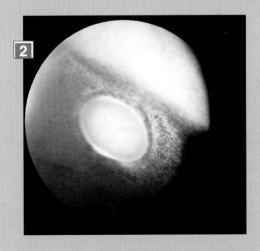

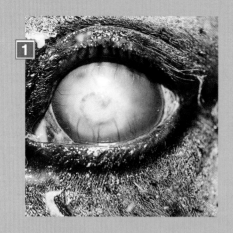

The eye in photo 1 has a central corneal ulcer caused by a fungal infection; note the blood vessels which have grown in from the edges to the site of the infection; the eye in photo 2 has a corneal ulcer infected with *Pseudomonas*, whose hallmark is the greenish hue to the lesion; the eye in photo 3 has an ulcer in the lower cornea caused by a foreign body imbedded in the third eyelid.

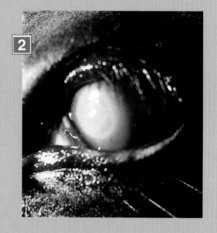

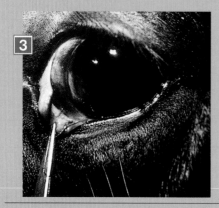

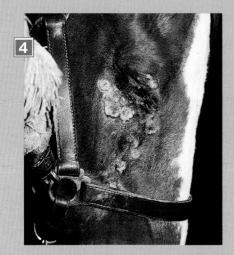

The eye in photo 4 has a fungal infection that is in the early stages; a microscopic view (photo 5) of material collected from an eye infected with a fungus growing in the corneal tissue; the eye in photo 6 is severely infected with *Pseudomonas* bacteria. It is characterized by a rapidly pro-gressing ulcer with a bluish-green tinge and a melting ap-pearance to the cornea.

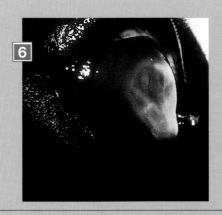

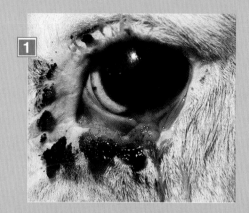

The horse in photo 1 has "cancer eye." The tumor "squamous cell carcinoma" occurs commonly in and around the eye, especially in horses with non-pigmented skin in this area.

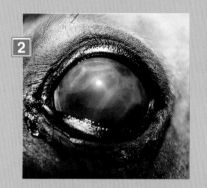
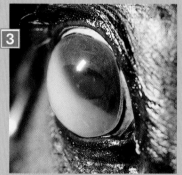

Photo 2 shows an eye suffering from glaucoma. As the eye swells from increased pressure, the inner layer of the cells of the cornea separate and cause the lines of edema noted, while the general increase in pressure causes the more generalized corneal edema; the eye in photo 3 is affected with corneal edema. If the outer surface of the cornea is damaged or the inner layer of cells become dysfunctional, the inner layer of the cornea absorbs water and develops the classic bluish, ground glass appearance. This particular case was caused by blunt trauma and hence the linear demarcation of the edema across the eye.

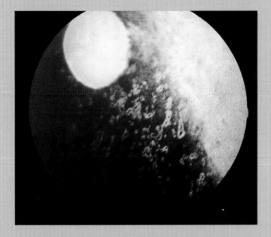

A view of the back of the eye as seen with the aid of the
ophthalmoscope; the mottled white areas scattered about
the pigmented fundus (the area surrounding the optic disc)
are scars, most likely blind spots, that resulted from
inflammation in the back of the eye

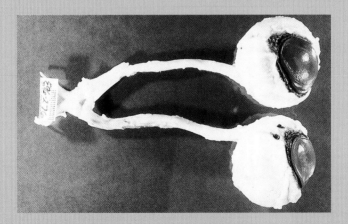

This is a pair of eyes that have been dissected from the
head. Note the optic nerves leading back to the optic
"chiasm" where the nerve signals cross over and go to
opposite sides of the brain.

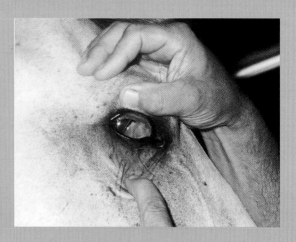

Checking the third eyelid, an anatomical structure that sweeps across the surface of the eye when the lids blink, acting like a windshield wiper to remove dust and debris and spreading the tear film across the corneal surface; the great racehorse Cigar and his "walleye."

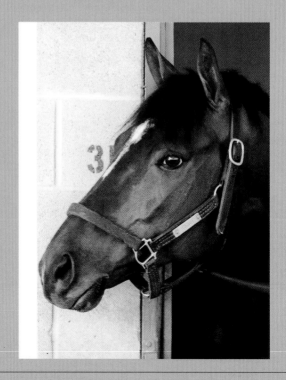

CORNEAL DISEASE

As mentioned in Chapter 4, the most common types of corneal disease involve ulceration and infection by bacteria or fungus. The initial corneal damage generally is caused by some form of trauma which opens the door for infection. In addition, there can be corneal lacerations which may require surgery to repair. The presence of foreign bodies lodged in the cornea after some type of trauma is not uncommon. The foreign bodies are typically some type of plant material. I have seen a foal that had a small piece of its mother's tail hair embedded in the cornea. Most of these foreign bodies can be "flushed" out of the cornea. Occasionally, the horse with a corneal foreign body will require surgery for its removal. In addition to bacterial and fungal infections of the cornea, there is a growing amount of evidence to support viral infections causing keratitis (or fungal infection) in the horse's eye.

CATARACTS

A cataract is essentially an opacity within the lens that interferes with the light's passage through the lens. A small cataract might not affect vision much, but a diffuse and dense one can block the light and cause blindness.

Cataracts can result from chronic uveitis, glaucoma, ocular trauma, and unknown causes. There are also congenital cataracts observed in foals. Unlike people, the horse does not suffer from diabetes, so that cannot be considered a cause.

Cataracts can be removed surgically in foals, and the horses tend to do well as adults. In adults, surgery is much more difficult because of the size of the eye, and it tends to have a poor outcome. In addition, cataracts in adults typically are caused by other advanced eye diseases that often have a poor prognosis anyway. Most cataracts can be seen easily with a flashlight, and usually the only question is how much vision has been affected.

THE BLOCKED DUCT

Remember the nasolacrimal duct from the anatomy section? This is the structure that runs from the two drainage holes in the corners of the eyes down through the skull and that opens up just inside the nostril. If you take a flashlight and look up a horse's nostril, focusing on the floor of the nasal passage about 2 to 3 inches up, you'll see a small pink defect in the tissue — this is the opening to the nasolacrimal duct. Chronic discharge from one or both eyes is a sign of a blocked nasolacrimal duct. To determine whether a duct is obstructed, veterinarians put a small amount of greenish-yellow dye into the eye and wait five to 10 minutes. If the duct is open, the dye will appear in the nostril.

Obstruction of a duct might be caused by swelling due to allergies, but there are other causes. If there is a defect in the bone (perhaps from a kick in the pasture), the duct might be affected where it passes through the bone. A chronic sinus infection or tumor also could affect the bone. Other possible factors could be an inflammation in the eye, such as conjunctivitis.

It is important to rule out other causes for a chronic eye discharge, which is why a complete ophthalmic examination is warranted. There might be an ulcer or other problem, such as a foreign body or tumor in the third eyelid.

If the blocked duct is the primary problem or secondary to a minor problem, the duct can be cleared. The doctor will place a catheter into the nasolacrimal opening in the nostril and flush it with saline. Only a veterinarian should perform this procedure because the duct is delicate; too much pressure can damage it and lead to significant problems.

ABNORMAL HAIRS AROUND THE EYE

We have already discussed "entropion" where the eyelids turn in (typically a disease in foals) and cause ulceration of the cornea from the abrasion. There occasionally can be growth of other abnormal hair fibers from the tissue surrounding the eye. These abnormal hairs can irritate the cornea, leading to possible ulcer development. The treatment for these abnormal hairs involves the removal of the tissue surrounding the hair fiber. The hair cannot just be plucked as it usually just grows back.

DERMOIDS

There is an abnormality of the eyeball surface called a "dermoid." A dermoid is a tumor-like structure that is an abnormal growth composed of skin, hair, and connective-type tissue. The effect on vision depends on the location of the lesion; those involving the cornea have the greatest impact. Treatment involves the surgical removal of the lesion; the outcome depends on the lesion's size and location and the success of surgery. If the dermoid involves large portions of the cornea, removal can lead to substantial scarring and therefore poor prognosis.

NIGHT BLINDNESS

Night blindness is often confused with moon blindness (uveitis), but it is a very different disease caused by a different problem — a deficiency of vitamin A.

The cells in the retina responsible for low-light vision are dependent on adequate concentrations of vitamin A to function properly, so a deficiency will lead to problems with low-light vision. It also can lead to blindness in the young horse. Without enough vitamin A, the canal of bone through which the optic nerve travels on its way to the brain will not grow properly. As the optic nerve enlarges, the canal is too small; subsequent pressure on the nerve causes it to die, leading to blindness. It's another good argument for eating carrots!

THE SUMMER SORE

Summer sores are technically called habronemiasis after the parasite *Habronema* which causes the problem. The larvae of the *Habronema* worm can infect tissue and cause a granular-looking lesion virtually anywhere on the body, including the soft tissue surrounding the eye. The lesions can be mistaken for some types of cancer or sarcoids. Careful examination and/or some laboratory examination can differentiate the problem. The treatment for habronemiasis involves deworming the animal. The deworming protocol should be devised by your veterinarian, who also should evaluate the lesion to rule out ocular cancer.

DRY EYE

A condition which sometimes affects horses but more commonly strikes dogs is "dry eye" in which the tissue that normally produces the tear film stops production. Remember that the tear film consists of different layers that function in protecting the eye. The tear film especially protects the surface of the cornea from drying out. In cases in which tear film production is reduced, the cornea is prone to dehydration, which in turn predisposes it to ulceration and subsequent infection. The disease can be treated with certain pharmaceuticals and the use of artificial tears.

SPECIAL PROBLEMS OF THE NEONATE

The foal is plagued with a few eye problems associated with being a baby. The most common is entropion (pronounced en-trop-ion), a condition in which the eyelashes roll inward and rub the cornea. The problem is most common in newborns (especially when premature) and causes intense irritation, ulceration, and potentially serious infection of the cornea. The condition can easily go unnoticed, so it is important to examine a newborn foal's eyes, especially if the eyes are being held closed. If you suspect the condition, DO NOT try to correct it by cutting off the lashes; the stubble will cause even more serious corneal injury. The problem can be corrected through minor surgery involving a few sutures or staples adjacent to the lid.

Another problem seen in foals is trichiasis (tri-chi-a-sis), a condition in which a normal eyelash goes in an abnormal direction (typically into the eye). The lash can cause irritation and corneal ulceration. Treatment consists of simply trimming the rogue eyelash.

The presence of congenital cataracts has been been discussed earlier in this book. In addition, the foal is subject to many of the eye diseases described here, including bactcrial and fungal ulcers.

Also, if a neonate develops a systemic blood infection from failure of passive transfer (it fails to ingest enough good quality colostrum during its first 24 hours), it often will develop an eye infection. The iris has a lot of blood vessels and perhaps acts as a filter for the bacteria. The iris can develop a greenish hue, and fibrin (an inflammatory protein) is present in the anterior chamber. Eye infections also are a complication of neonatal septicemia.

In addition, I have seen foals with various bodies lodged in the cornea (wood splinters and straw are some of the common culprits). In one case I found a small piece of tail hair, presumably from mom giving him a swish in the face.

CHAPTER 8

Systemic Diseases and the Eye

A number of systemic diseases and viruses can manifest in eye problems, ranging from dilated blood vessels in the eye to conjunctivitis and ocular discharge. Following are some of those diseases.

ENDOTOXIC SHOCK

Endotoxic shock or endotoxemia can be caused by numerous systemic diseases and most often is associated with gastrointestinal disturbances. Colics involving twisted intestine, or diarrheal diseases caused by Salmonella, can trigger endotoxemia. Toxins are produced in the blood stream, resulting in low blood pressure and subsequent cardiovascular deficiency. The low blood pressure is caused by a dilation of the blood vessels.

One of the clinical signs of endotoxemia is the presence of dilated and tortuous blood vessels in the sclera (white part) of the eye. The eye often is examined for signs of an increase in blood vessels (called sclera "injection") to confirm endotoxemia. In advanced cases of endotoxic shock, the blood vessels actually can start to leak and hemorrhage. This state is called DIC or disseminated intravascular coagulation and is considered grave. The hemorrhages usually are seen in the back of the eye around the fine blood vessels that surround the optic nerve.

DEHYDRATION SHOCK

The eye can reflect hydration status. As severe dehydration develops, tear secretions decrease and the surface of the cornea starts to take on a dry appearance. In addition, as the water in the tissue behind the eyes disappears, the eyes take on a sunken look as they sit back farther in the socket. The dry, sunken-eyed state is a sign of advanced dehydration.

AT A GLANCE

- Ocular problems can be signs of other diseases.

- An increase in blood vessels in the eye can indicate diseases such as endotoxemia, strangles, or EVA.

- EPM and other neurological diseases as well as certain cancers can result in blindness.

STRANGLES

Strangles is a disease that is caused by the bacterium *Streptococcus equi* and primarily affects the lymph nodes in the head. I occasionally have seen horses in which the lymph nodes in the ocular area are involved. In such cases, swollen lymph nodes cause the eye to bulge slightly out of the socket. There also may be an associated ocular discharge. An immune mediated disease associated with the strangles infection is called "purpura." Purpura inflames the blood vessels; in addition to causing swollen legs it can be seen in the eye as small hemorrhages of the blood vessels in the sclera or back of the eye.

EQUINE VIRAL ARTERITIS

Equine viral arteritis is a viral disease that causes an inflammation of the blood vessels. This virus can cause a variety of clinical signs ranging from reproductive problems such as sponta-

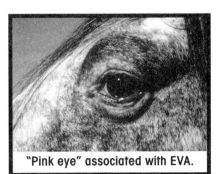
"Pink eye" associated with EVA.

neous abortion to respiratory disease. With certain forms of the disease, the eyes can show an increase in the blood vessels in the sclera (scleral injection), conjunctivitis, and ocular discharge. These ocular signs generally are accompanied by fever, swelling in the legs, and some form of respiratory disease.

EQUINE PROTOZOAL MYELOENCEPHALITIS

Equine protozoal myeloencephalitis (EPM) is a neurological disease caused by a protozoan parasite that infects the spinal column and the brain. The disease generally causes lameness or various gait abnormalities, but occasionally the parasite hits parts of the brain that control vision. If this occurs, the vision deficit depends on the site of the lesion. A lesion could affect vision only partially in one eye or both, or could cause a complete loss of sight.

OTHER NEUROLOGIC DISEASE

In addition to rabies, other neurologic viruses such as eastern/western encephalomyelitis and Venezuelan Equine Encephalomyelitis can cause blindness as one of their presenting signs. As far as other neurologic conditions, virtually anything that affects the areas of the brain that have control over vision can cause some degree of blindness.

Solitary tumors (either cancer or abscesses) can affect vision. Remember that the optic nerve crosses over so the left side of the brain responds to the right eye and the right side of the brain to the left eye. In very advanced types of pituitary tumors blindness can result. The pituitary gland is located just above where the optic nerves connect and cross over; the optic nerve is squashed against the floor of the skull by the enlarging pituitary tumor.

THE HERPES VIRUS

There are four known herpes viruses that cause disease in the horse. The one that causes upper respiratory disease also can cause conjunctivitis and ocular discharge. There is also some evidence that one of the herpes viruses can cause disease of the cornea. This viral type of keratitis (inflammation of the cornea) occurs in cats and most likely does occur in the horse.

RABIES

Rabies is a viral disease that is often passed on to the horse by the bite of an infected animal (usually a skunk or raccoon). Rabies is a fatal disease, and the affected horse typically dies within three days of the start of clinical signs. The clinical signs vary. A distinguished veterinary professor of mine often said, "The only predictable thing about rabies is that it is unpredictable." The

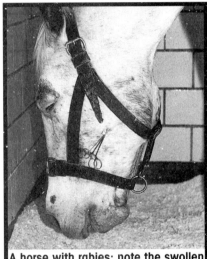

A horse with rabies; note the swollen eyelid.

virus causes an inflammation of the brain and the horse can present with either extreme depression or extreme rage. In addition, blindness can develop during the course of the disease.

SEPTICEMIA (NEONATAL)

As discussed previously, a foal with a blood infection can develop inflammation inside the eye. This is typically seen as a greenish coating on the iris and production of cotton candy-like fibrin in the anterior chamber.

JAUNDICE

Jaundice or icterous means a yellowing of the white part of the eye (sclera). Jaundice can be a clinical sign of a variety of illnesses. It is a classic sign of liver failure or certain kinds of blood disease.

The red blood cell normally is broken down in the body at a very slow rate, with one of the byproducts of this breakdown being a chemical called bilirubin. The bilirubin is processed by the liver and eliminated from the body via the gastrointestinal system. When the destruction of red blood cells is increased beyond the ability of the liver to process the bilirubin, there is a build up of bilirubin in the blood and it collects in the skin and other tissues, causing a yellowing. This is most prominent in the whites of the eyes.

One such blood disease is caused by red maple leaf toxicity. The ingestion of red maple leaves (especially if they are wilted) causes the destruction of red blood cells. Sometimes this disease is so rapid in course the horse dies before jaundice appears. Another blood disease is neonatal isoeurotholysis or NI. The NI condition occurs in foals when there is a reaction between the antibodies in the colostrum (the mare's first milk) and the baby's red blood cells, causing the destruction of those cells. Depending on the severity, this disease can occur so rapidly the foal dies before the jaundice is observed.

Jaundice can be observed with pure liver disease in the horse. Hepatitis (inflammation of the liver) can be caused by infection which will lead to jaundice. Hepatitis also can be caused by toxins such as Aslike clover or Fiddleneck (*Amsinckia*), Groundsel (*Senecio*), or Crotolaria. The ingestion of liver-toxic plants is usually a slow and chronic problem, so jaundice is typically observed with these toxicities. If there is an obstruction of the duct that moves the bilirubin into the gastrointestinal system, there can be a back up into the blood stream and jaundice will be observed. Remember that horses do not have a gallbladder, so they do not get gallstones (a cause of jaundice in people), but they can get an obstructed duct from intestinal twists and impactions.

Failure to eat is another cause of jaundice in the horse. The jaundice of fasting is a well-documented cause of yellow sclera and can occur at times of stress, colic, and numerous other diseases that put a horse off feed for several days. I have seen horses get the jaundice of fasting after long transports (New York to Florida, or shipping to Europe).

CHAPTER 9

First Aid, Care, and Maintenance

The most important aspects of first aid for the eye are prevention and awareness so problems can be detected as early as possible.

Horse owners' goals should try to prevent ocular accidents by eye-proofing their animals' environments. Go on a relentless search to find and remove anything that might injure the eye — nails, staples, tacks, wood splinters, etc. At horse shows, for instance, a stall might have been used as a tack room and could be loaded with potential weapons.

Hay racks and hay nets in the stall also put too much debris in the eye. The horse evolved eating at ground level, and that is the best place for it to eat.

The trailer is another place that can stress the eyes. If trips are short (less than four hours), don't ship horses with hay bags. If there is adequate ventilation in the trailer, the hay will blow around, and a lot of it will end up in the eyes. This is also hard on the respiratory system because horses inhale much of the airborne hay dust and particles. Trailer ventilation should be good, but indirect; drafts should not blow directly into a horse's face.

The goal is to find hazards before they find the horse's eye. The few minutes it takes to look around can save on vet bills and, in some cases, save a horse's eyeball.

Another good preventive measure is to leave a horse's facial hair alone. This includes not only the eyelashes and longer guard hairs around the eye, but the hair on the muzzle, which serves as a protective device. Some show people disagree, but there has been more than one A-circuit blue ribbon winner with all that hair still intact.

It is also important just to pay

> ## AT A GLANCE
>
> • Take steps to "eye-proof" your horse's environment.
>
> • Evaluate your horse's eyes on a daily basis and monitor for signs of pain.
>
> • Fly masks are useful as long as they fit properly.
>
> • Never medicate an eye without consulting a veterinarian.

attention to your horse's eyes. They should be evaluated daily and monitored for signs of pain, excessive tearing, or cloudiness.

I once was called to look at a horse that had developed "tumors" on the iris. The horse had been with its owner for three years, and the owner had been involved with horses for a long time. When I arrived, I was shown the "nigra" bodies, which had been there since birth.

Learn what the normal eye for your horse looks like. Take a penlight and check it out. By doing this several times, it will be easier to spot a problem should it arise. Consult your veterinarian if you notice anything abnormal.

Squinting or an ocular discharge, for example, is not normal, so don't write them off to "fly irritation" or something else.

FLY MASKS

Fly season can be hard on horses because the eyes seem to be a favorite target. But be extremely careful when using fly repellents because most of them can cause serious eye irritations. Never spray around the head; instead, put fly repellent on a towel and wipe it on the face, taking great care not to get any in the eyes.

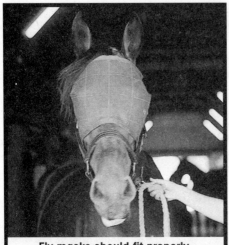
Fly masks should fit properly.

Ointment forms of repellents can be dangerous, too. On hot and sweaty days, they can melt and run into the eyes. And when using plastic repellent tags that attach to halters, be careful not to get them too close to the eye; the tags can cause a great deal of irritation. This also goes for liniments in bath water. Many of the bathing braces/liniments can cause ocular irritation, so be careful when washing the face.

Fly masks have become very popular. Like most things, however, they can cause problems for some horses, so be sure to get the correct size and adjust it properly. The stiff ones that form a cone over the eye can get pushed inward so the mask rubs on the eye and causes an ulcer. The net and stiffer mesh types can slip or, if too loose, allow flies to get in. The masks can work well, but they require some attention.

The other thing to remember is to "DO NO HARM." You should not self-medicate an eye with a potential problem. There are many types of eye ointments, and the wrong one could do a great deal of harm. Also, do not put anything in the eye that was not designed for that purpose. I once consulted on a case in Texas. The horse had had a runny eye for several weeks, and the owner, knowing there are a lot of fungal diseases in Texas, was spraying Jock Itch in the eye every day. The intention was good, but it was the wrong thing to do.

The best first aid is to prevent, notice problems early, and seek veterinary evaluation as soon as possible.

MEDICATION APPLICATION

The application of medication to the horse eye can be difficult at best. Most of the time your veterinarian will try to dispense an ointment in a small tube, but certain drugs only come in the form of drops, which are significantly more difficult to put in. The application of either an ointment or drop is a two-person job in most cases. Before application of the medication, the skin surrounding

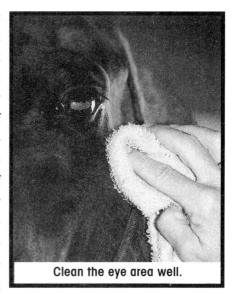

Clean the eye area well.

the eye should be gently cleaned with a cleansing material and warm water. This will remove any crusted discharge, which may attract flies. It also helps to relax the horse. If the eye has been painful and the horse has been getting treated multiple times per day for a period of time, the horse quickly will learn to resent treatment and anything you do to help it relax will make treatment easier.

Be careful to stand off to the side while treating the horse; you don't want to be in the strike zone if the horse decides to lash out with a front foot. The tip of the tube or dropper should be wiped off with a clean cloth prior to and after treatment. In addition, care should be taken not to touch the tip of the applicator with your fingers. Also, keep track of the applicator's lid; dirt can easily contaminate it.

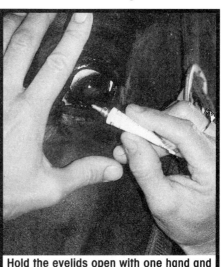

Hold the eyelids open with one hand and apply the medication with the other.

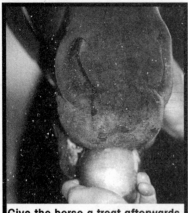

Give the horse a treat afterwards.

Have your handler hold the horse with its head tilted slightly to present the bad eye to you. The eyelids should be held open with one hand and the drug applied with the other. Be extremely careful not to poke the eye or even touch the surface of the cornea with the tip of the applicator. It will make future treatments easier if you spend some time comforting the horse and even giving it a treat after drug application.

Keep in mind that every ocular problem is different. There is a basic understanding of the various problems, but every case seems to respond differently to treatment. The most important thing to take away from this book is an understanding of what the normal eye looks like (especially for your individual horse) and what to look for if something is going wrong.

SOME FINAL WORDS

Should you have the misfortune to own a horse that ends up with some sort of visual problem, I would like offer the words of my mentor, Dr. William C. Rebhun. "Client education for the visually handicapped horse: Each horse with less than normal vision must be treated as an individual case when counseling owners concerning its usage. It must be realized that racing animals often must attempt to continue to perform to realize economic gains for the owners unless they have breeding potential. Many Standardbred racehorses and, to a lesser extent, Thoroughbred horses can actually race with rather severe visual handicaps. Those owners have to be aware of the animal's limitations; if the visual handicap results in balking, shying, breaking, or other abnormal behavior, racing will not be possible.

"For the pleasure of the performance horse, the question of visual soundness is extremely important. The higher the level of performance expected from the horse, the less visual handicap can be tolerated. In addition, the age and experience of the rider are of utmost importance since the visually imperfect horse may, at any time, show abnormal behavior or "spook" and the rider must be prepared to control a frightened, unpredictable animal. Therefore, a small child would not be a suitable rider for the average horse with limited vision. Many tractable horses that have adjusted to their visual handicap continue to be able to perform as trail horses or at other tasks not requiring total vision when guided by experienced riders."

FREQUENTLY ASKED QUESTIONS

HEALTH CONCERNS

How do I know if my horse is having a vision problem?

Some of this depends on whether the vision problem is sudden or slow brewing (as well as the individual animal). I have looked at some horses which are better than 75% blind, but lose their sight gradually over many months and you would hardly notice that they are having a vision problem. For the horse who is more troubled by loss of sight, the signs can be quite variable. If only one eye is affected, the horse can present with a strong degree of one-sidedness. Such a horse might crowd you in the stall when you are on the affected side. The horse might make radical head movements trying to keep you in the line of sight at all cost. When turned out, it could bump into objects or be very difficult to lead. Head shaking also can be a sign of certain vision problems.

In addition, the horse may not want to walk into strange places or small, confined areas. Also, these signs might worsen when the animal is out of its normal environment. As you can see, the signs are variable and depend on the individual horse and the specifics of its vision deficit. Many of these signs can be those of a troubled or poorly disciplined horse or the result of another medical problem, requiring an ophthalmic examination to determine the cause.

When should I be concerned about discharge from my horse's eye?

Basically any time there is discharge from the eye(s) there is cause for concern. The degree of concern depends on what the rest of the eye looks like. If the eye is painful (as indicated by squinting), there is a greater need for concern. Also, if there is a change in the surface of the cornea (cloudy or the presence of a bluish/white spot), it is a sign that the discharge may be a result of trauma or infection to the cornea.

The inside of the eye must be taken into consideration. If there is any haziness, there is likely to be inflammation or uveitis. If the third eyelid is protruding somewhat, there may be a problem associated with that structure causing the discharge. In addition, if it is in the middle of winter (the fly season long over) a discharge is likely to indicate a more serious problem. Sometimes ocular problems are manifestations of a systemic disease, so if the animal is off feed, has a fever, is acting lethargic, or is showing any other signs of illness, they could be related. If there is none of the above going on and the discharge is related to some other ocular irritation, seek veterinary consultation if the discharge persists for more than three days.

My horse has a sore eye with some discharge. I have some ointment left over from a problem my dog had (or I had). Is it safe to use that ointment on my horse?

This happens frequently and should NEVER be done. There are about 25 different ointments available for the treatment of ocular diseases. Most of the drugs are marketed for use in people and are used on animals in an "off-label" fashion. Species react differently to the same medication. If the horse has a corneal ulcer and is treated with an antibiotic ointment containing a steroid (used for anti-inflammatory properties) chances increase that it will develop a fungal infection. Fungal infections are bad and you do not want to encourage one. If an eye problem such as uveitis requires treatment with a steroid, monitor the condition of the eye diligently. Any ocular medication should be administered only on the advice of your veterinarian.

What's that white spot on my horse's cornea?

You need to consider what is going on with the rest of the eye. If the eye is painful and/or there is a discharge, there is a good chance that it is edema in the center of a corneal ulcer. Remember, any time the outer protective layer of the cornea is disrupted, water from the tears will soak into the inner layers of the cornea and create a bluish/white defect. In this case, your veterinarian should be consulted as soon as possible. If the eye appears healthy otherwise, there still can be an infection brewing in the case of a so-called stromal abscess. It also could be a defect on the inner surface of the cornea where the edema is coming from inside the eye (the aqueous). There is a chance that it is an old corneal scar (typically a dense white spot) that has been there for a long time and for whatever reason you are just noticing it now. If there is any question, consult your veterinarian.

What does a "blocked duct" mean?

The nasolacrimal duct is a structure that runs from the eye to the tip of the nostril. If you look inside the nostril, you will see a small pink hole just beyond the normal line of sight. That's the opening to the duct. Its function is to drain the tears. If the duct becomes inflamed or occluded (blocked) from some sort of trauma to the skull bone (the middle portion of the duct travels through the skull), there will be a chronic ocular discharge. If the condition is chronic, the eye's environment will change and conjunctivitis might develop. In addition, if there is some other ocular disease such as uveitis or an ulcer, the duct can become occluded as a secondary problem and remain so long after the primary problem has been resolved. In such cases, the duct needs to be "flushed." The procedure is generally performed under light sedation or with the application of some sort of restraint. (I have found the "Stabilizer" to be a superior method of restraint for this procedure.) When the horse is ready, a catheter is threaded into the nostril, then a saline solution is "flushed" through to clear the blockage; the saline will come out the eye. This procedure should only be performed by your veterinarian, as the duct is sensitive and can be damaged if the flush pressure is too great.

Should an eye exam be part of a pre-purchase exam?

An ocular examination is a very important part of the routine pre-purchase examination. The purpose of the purchase examination is to determine if the horse in question is sound for its intended use. For some divisions of competition governed by the American Horse Shows Association, the lack of vision is considered an unsoundness and would therefore prohibit a horse with a vision problem from showing. For the racehorse, depending on which state you are going to race in, it may not be a problem (if it is not a problem for the horse).

Another important aspect of the pre-purchase examination and the eye examination is to try to detect the presence of old (inactive) signs of moon blindness or uveitis. Scars in the back of the eye (on the retina) surrounding the optic disc can indicate this condition and require examination with the ophthalmoscope to see. The importance of this is that uveitis is a recurring disease, so in addition to potentially affecting vision on the day of the examination, it could become a problem in the future. This is a difficult one because it is a very unpredictable disease and may come back next week or never. In addition, if it recurs it could be mild or severe and there is no way to predict its severity.

My horse's eye needs to be removed. Is it the end of the world?

In most cases, the removal of a horse's eye is far more traumatic to the owner than to the horse. Most horses adapt extremely well to the loss of one eye. In fact, I have seen many cases where chronic pain caused by a long-standing ocular problem has led to eye removal. In these cases, the horse's demeanor improved significantly after surgery, most likely due to the sudden reduction in pain. The procedure is usually performed under general anesthesia and takes 30 to 45 minutes. The eye is removed and the lids are sutured together. There is an adjustment period, but for many horses the vision in the affected eye has been substantially reduced and they have already adapted to one-eyed sight. It takes longer for the owner and those involved with the horse to become accustomed to the loss of the eye.

With some show horses, the American Horse Shows Association considers the loss of sight in one eye an "unsoundness" and these horses no longer can compete. Check with the AHSA to see if your horse falls in this category. Many performance horses continue to do well despite the loss of one eye. Some states permit a one-eyed horse or a horse that is blind in one eye to race. Special permission is required to ensure that the horse has adapted well and is not a danger to the jockey or the other horses. So if your horse has the misfortune to lose an eye, it is not the end of the world.

ANATOMY AND GENETICS

What are the brown bag-like structures on the iris?

It is amazing how many horse owners go for years without noticing these little structures and then one day see them and panic, thinking something is drastically wrong. The structures are called the copra nigra or nigra bodies. They are a perfectly normal part of the anatomy of the equine eye. Their function is unknown, but many veterinarians have hypothesized that they act as some sort of sun shade. Occasionally they can be quite large and even become cyst-like, filling up a large part of the anterior chamber. In such cases, they are obscuring vision and need to be reduced surgically. When the nigra bodies become fluid-filled cysts, they are reduced by inserting a syringe needle and aspirating the fluid.

Why do some horses have a white ring around their eyes?

Well, because that's the way it is. Not a very scientific explanation, but... This condition has halted the sale of many a nice horse just because the white ring has a bad rap. The condition is referred to as "walleyed" and is one of the many genetic variations these wonderful animals have. There is a great deal of folklore surrounding this variation of normal — most of it bad. These horses often are claimed to be poor performers, plagued with unsoundness, maniacal in behavior, and just plain trouble. None of these problems has ever been proven to be connected with the white ring and there are plenty of nut case horses without the white ring. Also, there are some great performance horses (and some very lovable ponies) that have this infamous white ring. Cigar, the leading earner among Thoroughbred racehorses of the 20th Century, has a walleye.

Is a light-colored iris normal?

The vast majority of horses have a brown iris. But occasionally you will see a horse with a bluish/white or even greenish-colored iris. This is a normal (but somewhat rare) variation and does not affect the horse's vision. As with the walleyed horse, the horse with the unusually colored iris gets a bad rap as some horse people equate it with poor performance, poor health, and/or a predisposition to eye problems. But this is not the case.

Can horses see in the dark?

Horses, based on the inner anatomy of the eye and observation, can see in the dark better than people can. Remember that they (as well as many other creatures) have the tepetium lecuidum, which is the layer of cells in the back of the eye that reflects light. This is what you see when the car's headlights spy out some little creature or a deer on the side of the road. Of course, they need some light, but a bright, star-filled sky or a clear moon probably gives ample light for those nocturnal wanderings in the paddock. But until horses talk or we learn to talk horse, to what extent they really see in low light conditions will remain a mystery.

COMFORT AND SAFETY

Should I use a fly mask on my horse?

There is nothing more pitiful than a horse out at pasture during the summer with its face coated with flies that suck away at the ocular fluids (and spread disease while they are at it). Fly masks were a good invention and can make a real difference. You must be careful with them so that they don't cause a problem. Make sure that you get the right size and fit it to your horse properly. An ill-fitting mask actually can rub the eye and cause an ulcer. Check on the horse frequently to make sure that the mask is not in the eye. I also have seen ill-fitting masks that allow flies to get underneath, causing the horse to go bonkers.

There are some repellent ointments available for use around the eyes. Take great care not to get any of the fly sprays in the eye. On a really hot and humid day, the ointments or spray/wipes can run into the eye with the sweat and burn the cornea. I also have seen eye injuries related to the plastic tags that are attached to the halter —make sure that they do not come into contact with the eye.

Can I safely trim the whiskers around the eyes for cosmetic reasons?

In my opinion: no, no, and no. All of the hairs surrounding the eyes, especially the lashes, are there as part of the eye's self-defense system. If you trim any of these, you will greatly increase the risk of ocular trauma.

Is there anything I can do to reduce the risk of eye injury?

Absolutely. You need to examine every inch of your horse's environment looking for that stray nail, staple, or piece of sheet metal. Check out all new stalls, especially at horse shows. Examine fence posts and trailers for protruding objects. I also have seen eye lacerations caused by sharp wire on electric fence connectors. Feed mangers in the pasture, as well as water devices, can have many sharp areas that need to be fixed. Make sure snaps used to hang feed and water buckets face inward so your horse's eye is protected as it sticks its head into the bucket.

I believe that hay racks and nets increase the risk of ocular problems (and possibly respiratory problems as well). Horses evolved to eat off of the ground and that is how they should be fed. Unless you are shipping your horse a great distance, I do not recommend shipping with a hay net because of hay dust and particles blowing into the horse's face. If you absolutely must ship with hay, the hay nets should be soaked in water to reduce the chaff blowing around.

While grooming, be careful not to get any debris in the eyes. Examine the eyes on a daily basis so you learn what the normal eye looks like and can spot a potential problem early.

CASE STUDIES

The following cases are based on actual situations I have encountered in my practice. They represent issues that confront horse owners and potential owners at various times.

CASE NO. 1 (UVEITIS)

The horse of your dreams is in hand and you are just waiting for the final word from me, your veterinarian, about the results of pre-purchase examination. I give you news that unfortunately raises more questions than it answers. That's because I have found a small but telltale lesion deep inside the eye that is indicative of a prior episode of uveitis. The ocular examination is a very important part of the routine pre-purchase examination and looks for any problems that might affect the horse's ability to perform. Remember that uveitis is an inflammatory condition affecting the interior of the eye and may cause scarring in the retinal area that can affect vision. A more important fact about uveitis or moon blindness is the fact that it can recur, hence one of its names: periodic ophthalmia.

This horse has a small lesion in the retinal area that appears as a small scar next to the optic disc. I determine that the scar probably isn't affecting vision significantly based on all other examination findings, the horse's history, and the character of the lesion. The question remains, what to do now? Based on what we know about the disease, it can recur and in severe cases lead to blindness. This horse is middle-aged and based on the history has not suffered from any obvious ocular disease within the last three years. However, there is the scar in the back of the eye. This is a difficult situation because I cannot predict what might happen — the disease might never recur, or the horse could suffer from a bout of ocular inflammation next week.

As with everything, we are usually biased by our past experiences. If you previously owned a horse that suffered from uveitis, you may not want to touch this horse with a 10-foot pole. On the other hand, you may decide this is an acceptable gamble if the horse is perfect in all other respects. Your veterinarian can tell you only the facts about what he or she finds in the eye on the day of the examination. That information can be useful in helping you reach the decision only you can make.

CASE NO. 2 (WRONG MEDICATION)

A middle-aged pleasure horse returns from a weekend trail ride with an irritated eye. The surrounding ocular tissue is slightly puffy, the conjunctiva red and irritated, the horse is squinting, and there is a stream of watery ocular discharge coming down the side of the face. The owner has some eye ointment in the barn's medicine cabinet left over from a horse that had an ocular problem a few months earlier and decides to treat the eye with this ointment for a few days. Initially the eye responds quite well to the ointment. The redness and the pain subside, then suddenly the irritation returns along with a small, cloudy spot on the cornea. This time the pain is extreme, with the horse barely opening the eye. The owner calls me.

On examination, I determine that the eye has a rapidly progressing corneal ulcer infected with a fungus. The eye has changed rapidly in a very short period of time with approximately 50% of the corneal surface being affected within a few days of the diagnosis. The necessary treatment requires application of a reasonably expensive antifungal drug every two hours around the clock; this extreme frequency of treatment is often required to control a serious corneal infection. The owner attempts to keep up the pace with treatments for several days on the farm, but soon burns out and chooses to have the horse hospitalized for treatment. The horse is treated every two hours for approximately three weeks — a long and expensive course of therapy.

The eye is saved, but the cornea remains scarred with a white spot about the size of a dime; the horse returns to training and actually performs well, despite some visual deficit due to the scarring. The horse's five weeks of hospitalization and treatment cost $5,000.

In reviewing the initial treatment, I determine that the eye was treated on the farm with an ocular ointment that contained a steroid. The ointment originally had been prescribed for a horse suffering from uveitis; the treatment of choice for uveitis is a steroid ointment. The use of a steroid containing ointment is not indicated for ocular diseases where there is the presence of a corneal ulcer due to the increased risk of developing a fungal infection. (Note: it may be necessary with uveitis, but it is a risk.) The steroids decrease the local immune defenses of the eye and predispose to the development of fungal disease.

Approximately 65% of horses I have treated with fungal eye disease had received prior treatment with a steroid ointment. In this case, the horse probably had a scratch on the cornea from trail riding. Although the eye responded well (initially) to the powerful anti-inflammatory effects of the topical steroid, it rapidly deteriorated as the fungal infection took hold. The ointment also contained an antibiotic, which potentially would have limited any bacterial infection, but not deter any fungal invaders.

In this case the indiscriminate use of a medication prescribed for a different animal was a costly mistake that could have (and has in other cases) resulted in blindness. For this very reason, no medication should ever be administered without veterinary consultation. Many drugs have the potential to do a great deal of harm depending on the individual circumstances, and their use should be taken very seriously.

CASE NO. 3 (CONGENITAL CATARACTS)

You are the proud owner of a newborn Thoroughbred foal. Everything seems to be all right, but the foal appears to have some trouble finding the milk supply. He does find the milk, but it takes a bit longer than other foals you have had in the past. The foal also appears to be a little extra spooky and nervous, especially when you reach out to touch him; he goes a little bonkers when you actually get a hand on him. On closer inspection, you note that the eyes appear to have a milky white color in the center where the rich and dark black pupil should be. You are getting the foal checked tomorrow as a matter of routine, and make a mental note

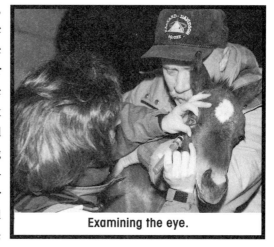

Examining the eye.

to ask your veterinarian about the milky color within the eyes.

At the time of examination, I take a close look at the pupil with a strong focal light source (a fancy flashlight). Already suspicious of congenital cataracts, I check the special reflection of light off of the lens. Remember that congenital means "to be born with" and that congenital cataracts do occur in the horse. Also remember that a cataract is defined as any opacity of the lens; it can be a small focal spot in just one eye resulting from uveitis or even trauma or a cataract can be diffuse and involve the entire lens on one or both sides. Congenital cataracts typically affect both eyes and are of a diffuse nature, making the entire lens opaque to various degrees. If the lens is opaque, the light that has passed through the cornea will hit the opacity in the lens and be reflected back, causing the white color or sparkle to be noted.

I conclude that the new foal has congenital cataracts and recommend surgery. If the cataract is not treated, the horse will grow up with a significant visual deficit. Cataracts in adult horses are more difficult to treat and have a worse prognosis (especially depending on what caused them), but in the foal the prognosis is actually relatively good. The surgery involves the same technique used in people, which is called phacoemulsification. Phaco means lens and to emulsify means stirring it up and turning it into a liquid. The lens in foals is softer and can be broken up more easily than in an adult. The process also is made easier because the lens actually is sort of like Jell-O inside a plastic sandwich bag; the lens is surrounded by a capsule.

The foal is placed under anesthesia and a needle is inserted into the eye and then into the lens. The outer capsule stays intact and the inner lens material is broken down. When the inner lens material is emulsified, it is sucked out of the lens capsule by the needle, effectively removing the opacified lens material.

How will the absence of a lens affect your foal's vision? Actually, very little. In the horse, most of the light entering the eye is bent and focused by the cornea. The lens, in a relative sense, does not contribute that much to focusing the light on the surface of the retina. Remember that if the light is not focused on the retina, the image will not be in focus either.

The foal in question had both cataracts removed by the above technique and is now grown up and a relatively nice performance horse. If you happen to find yourself owning a foal with congenital cataracts, it is not the end of the world. Just realize that surgical treatment is required and that the sooner surgery is performed the better the prognosis.

GLOSSARY

Aqueous flare — A phenomenon associated with uveitis where the aqueous humor in the anterior chamber has become cloudy due to the presence of white blood cells coming from the inflammation. When a light beam is projected into the eye the aqueous flare can be seen like a flashlight beam in a smoke-filled room.

Anterior — A directional term used for the front surface of the eye.

Anterior chamber — The space between the inner surface of the cornea and the anterior surface of the iris and lens.

Aqueous humor — The clear fluid that fills up the anterior chamber.

Bacterial keratitis — An ulcer or abscess of the cornea that is infected with a bacterium.

Blepherospasm — The hallmark of a painful eye; the horse squints.

Blocked duct — Any condition (usually inflammation) that occludes the nasolacrimal duct causing an ocular discharge.

Cancer eye — Squamous cell carcinoma affecting the eye or surrounding tissue (the third eyelid is a common location for this type of cancer).

Canthus — The area of the eyelids where the upper and lower meet; the medial and lateral canthus.

Cataract — Any opacity on any aspect of the lens.

Caudal — A directional term meaning on the back surface of the body.

Conjunctiva — The soft pink tissue lining the underside of the eyelids and surrounding the eye.

Conjunctivitis — An inflammation of the conjunctiva.

Cornea — The clear surface of the eye. The cornea bends light and causes it to focus on the back of the eye.

Corneal edema — A collection of water in the stroma causing a bluish/white discoloration of the cornea.

Cranial — A directional term meaning on the forward surface of the body.

Edema — A collection of water.

Endothelium — The posterior layer of cells on the inner surface of the cornea.

Entropion — The condition where the eyelashes roll inward and actually rub the corneal surface causing ulceration (generally a disease of foals).

Enucleation — The surgical process of removing one of the eyes.

Epiphora — The presence of an ocular discharge or excessive tearing.

Epithelium — The anterior layer of cells on the outer surface of the cornea.

Fibrin — Fibrin is one of the main proteins formed by inflammation and can be seen within the anterior chamber like mounds of cotton candy floating about as a result of various causes of inflammation; fibrin is a precursor to more mature scar tissue and can be quite damaging to the interior of the eye if left unchecked.

Focal point — The point at which the light being transmitted through the eye comes into focus; if the light comes into focus in front of or behind the retina, the image will be out of focus.

Fungal keratitis — An ulcer or abscess of the cornea that is infected with a fungus.

Glaucoma — A disease that is characterized by an increased pressure inside of the eye.

Hypopeon — A collection of white blood cells within the anterior chamber that form a white snow like layer on the floor of the chamber, most commonly associated with uveitis.

Hyphemia — A collection of blood within the eye typically from ocular trauma.

Icterous — A yellowing of the sclera caused by a variety of conditions.

Iris — The tissue (usually brown in the horse) surrounding the pupil that dilates or constricts depending on the intensity of the ambient light.

Iris cyst — The development of a cyst within the nigra bodies.

Jaundice — A yellowing of the sclera caused by a variety of conditions.

Keratitis — Inflammation of the cornea.

Keratomycosis — A fungal infection of the cornea.

Lacrimal glands — The gland tissue surrounding the eye that is responsible for manufacturing the tear film.

Lateral — A directional term meaning on the outside surface of the body.

Lens — The clear structure that occupies the space behind the iris; it is observed as the pupil.

Lens luxation — A condition in which the lens has been completely dislocated from its normal position behind the iris, generally a result of trauma.

Lens subluxation — A condition in which the lens is only partially dislocated from its normal position; a result of trauma or chronic uveitis.

Medial — A directional term meaning on the inside surface of the body.

Meiosis — A constriction of the pupil, making it smaller.

Mycosis — A fungal infection.

Mydriasis — A dilation of the pupil, making it bigger.

Nasal — A directional term meaning toward the nose.

Nasolacrimal duct — The duct that allows the drainage of tears from the eye to the lower aspect of the nostril.

Nigra bodies (corpora nigra) —The black punching-bag like structures (normally present in the horse) on the upper aspect of the iris.

Nystagmus — An abnormal movement of the eyes usually caused by a neurologic condition.

Optic disc — The white dot in the center of the retina which is the optic nerve entering the back of the eye.

Photophobia — A hypersensitivity to bright light (as noted by squinting) due to ocular pain.

Posterior — A directional term used for the back surface of the eye.

Puncta — The openings of the nasolacrimal duct on the inner surface of the lower eye lid.

Pupil — The black dot in the center of the iris caused by the dark reflection of the inner eye seen through the clear lens.

Retina — The receptor layer on the back surface of the eye that collects light and starts the process of converting it into an electrical signal to be sent to the brain via the optic nerve.

Sclera — The white tissue making up about 75% of the eye.

Scleral injection — An increase in the number of blood vessels within the sclera.

Stroma — The cells making up the inner portion of the cornea.

Stromal abscess — A tiny abscess within the stroma of the cornea usually caused by a small puncture- type wound to the cornea.

Synechia — The presence of scar tissue inside the eye. Synechia may go from the iris to the inner surface of the cornea, from the iris to the front surface of the lens, etc. It can prevent the movement of the iris in response to light, effectively gluing it down to other structures within the eye.

Tactile hair — The important hair (not the lashes) surrounding the eye; this hair should never be cut back due to the predisposition to ocular trauma if it is removed.

Temporal — A directional term meaning away from the nose.

Tepedum — The greenish/yellow reflective tissue in the upper portion of the back of the eye responsible for amplifying light in low light situations. This is the tissue responsible for the bright reflection a car's headlights make in the eyes of some nocturnal creatures.

Third eyelid — The flap of soft tissue under the nasal aspect of the lower eyelid that can act as a windshield wiper and sweep debris off of the corneal surface.

Ulcer — An area of the cornea that has the epithelium missing for a variety of reasons.

Uvea — All of the vascular tissue within the eye, especially lining the iris and surrounding tissue and the tissue underneath the retina.

Uveitis (periodic ophthalmia or moon blindness) — An inflammation of the uveal tissue within the eye.

Vitreous humor — The clear, jelly-like fluid that occupies the space between the posterior surface of the iris and lens and the retina.

Vitrial floater — The remains of cellular debris that can actually float around within the posterior chamber as the horse moves its head; these floaters can be an uncommon cause of head shaking or spooking.

INDEX

RECOMMENDED READINGS

Ball, MA. *Understanding Equine First Aid*. Lexington, KY:The Blood-Horse, Inc., 1998.

Ball, MA. *Understanding Basic Horse Care*. Lexington, KY:The Blood-Horse, Inc., 1999.

Barrett, KC et al. *Colour Atlas and Text of Equine Ophthalmology*. London: Mosby-Wolfe, 1995.

Blakely, J. *Horses and horse sense: the practical science of horse husbandry*. Reston, VA: Reston Publishing Company, Inc., 1981.

Robinson, NE. ed. *Current Therapy in Equine Medicine 4*. Philadelphia: W. B. Saunder Company, 1997.

Siegal, M. ed. *UC Davis Book of Horses*. New York: HarperCollins Publishers, Inc., 1996.

Equine Eye sites on the Internet

The Horse: Your Online Guide to Equine Health Care:
http://www.thehorse.com

American Association of Equine Practitioners:
http://www.aaep.org

The Hay.net's veterinary resources page:
http://www.haynet.net/Veterinary_Resources/

Equine Recurrent Uveitis: Information for the Horse Owner:
http://www.igs.net/~vkirkwoodhp/eru.htm

The Horseman's Advisor. Go to Equine Diseases: Eye Diseases:
http://www.horseadvice.com/advisor/

Antifungal Home. Dr. Michael A. Ball's review of fungal diseases
and drugs used to treat them:
http://www.people.cornell.edu/pages/mab20/

Picture Credits

CHAPTER 1
Anne M. Eberhardt, 12; Michael A. Ball, 12.

CHAPTER 3
Tom Hall, 28; Anne M. Eberhardt, 29.

CHAPTER 4
Tom Hall, 30, 35; Michael A. Ball, 31.

CHAPTER 5
Michael A. Ball, 40.

CHAPTER 6
Benoit & Associates, 44; Matt Goins, 45-46; Michael A. Ball, 46-47.

CHAPTER 7
Michael A. Ball, 49-55; Barbara D. Livingston, 56; Anne M. Eberhardt, 56.

CHAPTER 8
Dr. Peter Timoney, 63; Michael A. Ball, 65.

CHAPTER 9
Tom Hall, 70–72.

CASE STUDIES
Anne M. Eberhardt, 85.

EDITOR — JACQUELINE DUKE

ASSISTANT EDITOR — JUDY L. MARCHMAN

COVER/BOOK DESIGN — SUZANNE C. DEPP

ILLUSTRATIONS — ROBIN PETERSON

COVER PHOTO— ANNE M. EBERHARDT

About the Author

Michael A. Ball, DVM, a native of upstate New York, worked professionally in the horse industry for six years before earning a bachelor's degree in animal science from the College of Agriculture and Life Sciences at Cornell University

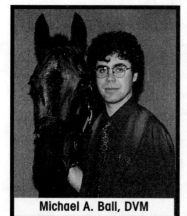

Michael A. Ball, DVM

and subsequently a degree in veterinary medicine, also from Cornell. After Cornell, he completed an internship in large animal medicine and surgery and also served as an instructor in the Department of Anesthesia at the University of Georgia.

After Georgia, Ball returned to Cornell and completed a residency in large animal internal medicine and the requirements for a Master of Science degree in pharmacology. He is board eligible with the American College of Veterinary Internal Medicine and the College of Veterinary Clinical Pharmacology.

Ball has served as a lecturer and clinician at Cornell. In additional to his academic pursuits in internal medicine and clinical pharmacology, Ball maintains a strong interest in clinical practice related to performance horses of all types and devotes a substantial effort to owner education on equine health issues. He is the author of *Understanding Equine First Aid* and *Understanding Basic Horse Care*, part of The Horse Health Care Library series, and a frequent contributor to *The Horse* magazine. He lives in Ithaca, N.Y., with his wife, Christina Cable, also a veterinarian.